WHAT HE CAN EXPECT WHEN SHE'S NOT EXPECTING

WHAT HE CAN EXPECT WHEN SHE'S NOT EXPECTING

HOW TO SUPPORT YOUR WIFE, SAVE YOUR MARRIAGE, AND CONQUER INFERTILITY!

MARC SEDAKA
With Gregory F. Rosen, M.D., F.A.C.O.G.

SKYHORSE PUBLISHING

All Rights Reserved. No part of this book may be reproduced in any manner without the express written consent of the publisher, except in the case of brief excerpts in critical reviews or articles. All inquiries should be addressed to Skyhorse Publishing, 307 West 36th Street, 11th Floor, New York, NY 10018.

Skyhorse Publishing books may be purchased in bulk at special discounts for sales promotion, corporate gifts, fund-raising, or educational purposes. Special editions can also be created to specifications. For details, contact the Special Sales Department, Skyhorse Publishing, 307 West 36th Street, 11th Floor, New York, NY 10018 or info@skyhorsepublishing.com.

Skyhorse® and Skyhorse Publishing® are registered trademarks of Skyhorse Publishing, Inc.®, a Delaware corporation.

www.skyhorsepublishing.com

10 9 8 7 6 5 4 3 2 1

Library of Congress Cataloging-in-Publication Data is available on file.

ISBN: 978-1-61608-058-7

Printed in the United States of America

For Samantha . . .

Who always knew better.

CONTENTS

FOREWORD

BY DR. GREGORY ROSEN, M.D.

Most of us were raised with the American credo that hard work will always produce the intended results, and, conversely, failure to achieve your goals only occurs when you haven't tried hard enough. Infertility, for some, is the first instance when the American credo fails.

My parents were told in the late 1940s that they would never have children, yet here I am typing out the foreword to Marc's book. Persistence was what helped them, because there was no technology for measuring hormones, no medications to take that could improve or cause ovulation. They didn't know about basal body temperature charting, and no one taught them about cervical mucus changes for coital timing. No one did inseminations or IVF, and the technology of ultrasound was still about 40 years away. Social and sexual taboos ruled medicine. It was thought to be always the female's problem, and my father never had a semen analysis, despite the fact that my mother had multiple X-rays of her uterus.

A sad but true story about my family occurred when I was still in medical school, and I was working with my parents in the backyard. I initially approached my mother, when my father was out of earshot, and asked her why they had had so much trouble having children. She told me that it was my father's fault. I asked her how she knew, and she stated that all the tests that had been done on her were all normal, and the doctors had refused to examine my father. A few minutes later, when out of earshot from my mother, I asked my father the same question. He told me that it was all my mother's fault! One of the many conversations I regret not having with my father before his death was why he thought he was not part of the problem.

Thankfully, men have come a long way since my father's time, and that's why a book like this is so long overdue. As Marc so smartly stresses, infertility is not a male issue or a female issue, it is a couple's issue. As a good husband, you are needed to do what men have been bred to do since Adam and Eve: listen to your wife, support your wife, and protect her when needed. (And, of course, *read this book!*)

Greg Rosen
January 2011

WHAT HE CAN EXPECT WHEN SHE'S NOT EXPECTING

INTRODUCTION

On January 29, 2003, I witnessed a miracle. At exactly 11:30 PM, my first child, Amanda Esther Sedaka, was born. Seventeen minutes later, my second child, Charlotte Dawn Sedaka, followed her sister into the world. Two beautiful baby girls, not even 10 pounds between them, had just gasped their first breaths.

This, however, was not the miracle.

The miracle was that the woman who delivered my daughters—one the spitting image of me, the other the spitting image of my wife—was, in fact, not my wife. She was what is called a gestational surrogate. In the simplest terms, she was a "womb for rent" who, nearly nine months earlier, had our then five-day-old embryos implanted inside her uterus.

God bless modern science!

Now keep in mind that hiring a gestational surrogate is not a decision one comes to lightly. I didn't just wake up one morning and say, "Hey, honey, here's a nutty idea. How's about we get ourselves one of those gestational surrogates to carry our kids for us?" Hell, a year before, I barely knew what either of those words meant.

Like anything else, having these babies was a process. One that, in the case of my wife and me, took us from "actively trying" to get pregnant, to fertility medication, to sixteen artificial inseminations, to nine in vitro fertilizations, to finally, the mother of all cutting-edge technological advancements to date—the aforementioned gestational surrogate. In all, six years, three states, five doctors, and $250,000. Yikes!

So why am I writing a book about it? (I mean, other then to scare the shit out of you?) Because as a guy who's been through the process and lived to tell about it, I know how frustrating and confusing the infertility journey can be—especially for the husband, whose role is so often ill defined and overlooked. You see, for all the support groups and self-help books and talk show segments geared toward the woman, there is very little infertility information aimed specifically toward the man. So more often than not, we poor schlubs are left to fend for ourselves—not quite sure when to chime in, when to keep quiet, when to take action, when to lay low. And rest assured, if you're anything like I was, you'll make the completely wrong decision every time.

This book is your opportunity to learn from my mistakes. It's written by a man, for a man, and, with that in mind, doesn't waste your precious time with lots of technical mumbo-jumbo or disturbing diagrams of the female anatomy. (Your wife probably has you reading about 20 of those books as it is.) Instead, we're going to stick to frank discussions, inappropriate references, and crude language whenever possible. In short, the kind of book I wish I had been forced to read when I was going through this hell—I mean, process.

Now, as you've probably guessed, the one potential drawback to reading a book written by a layman is that he may not always have all the answers—especially when it comes to trivial little details like medical knowledge and cold, hard facts. That's why I've enlisted the help of a world-renowned fertility doctor, the *incredibly* knowledgeable Dr. Gregory Rosen, to not only verify my information but also provide invaluable expert commentary whenever necessary.

So fasten your seat belt, take a deep breath, and prepare to enter a world you never, in all your wildest dreams, imagined you'd ever be a part of. I can't promise all the information will be pleasant (remember the quarter of a million dollars a few paragraphs back?), but at least it will be straightforward and honest. And with any luck, you'll come out the other side feeling that much more secure about whatever the hell it is you're supposed to be doing now.

MAPPING OUT YOUR INFERTILITY JOURNEY

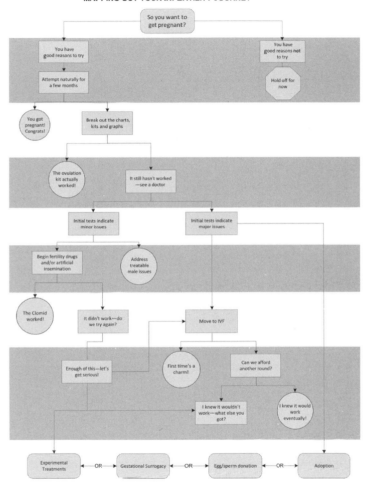

ROUND ONE
THE TRYOUTS

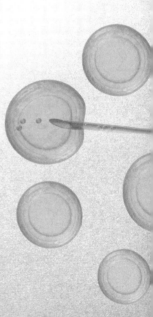

It was inevitable. At some point after getting married, one of us (and it sure as heck wasn't going to be me), was going to broach the subject of children—or, more specifically, when to have them. We were both 29 at the time, and my wife proposed that we wait a year and then actively try at 30. I countered with a less stringent and more pleasant-sounding "someday." We finally compromised on trying at 31 and a baby at 32.

So what was the end result? Trying at 30 (she got more than her way as usual), and babies (twins) at 36. Six years of trying! Something neither of us had taken into account, but a sad reality for far too many couples. Remember, *trying* to get pregnant and actually *getting* pregnant are two very different concepts, so don't assume that one will automatically lead to the other. For better or worse, this is one of those times where you're going to have to plan ahead . . . because there's honestly no telling how long the trying may take.

In this first section, we'll explore that critical "trying" time—when to start, when to take additional steps and, most important, how to avoid getting blamed for anything. (Because, in the end, isn't that what it's all about?) If this is where you are in the process, then read on. If not, feel free to skip right to Round II,

"Spring Training," where we begin to discuss the many procedures and treatments that you guys may be going through at this very moment. (Just make sure to rough up the next few pages a bit so she at least *thinks* you read them. See? It's all about covering your ass.)

1

WHEN TO START TRYING

Have you ever been to a fertility clinic's waiting room? If not, then allow me to set the stage. First of all, it's filled. Standing room only. The patients, mostly women, of course (with a handful of glassy-eyed husbands thrown in for good measure), sit solemnly—their eyes darting to and fro—silently sizing up the office, its staff, and, of course, their fellow sufferers. And the average age? I'm going to say 41. In fact, when my wife and I went to our first (of many) infertility specialists at age 32, we were easily the youngest people in the room!

Now, while I'm sure there were good reasons why many of these women waited as long as they did, I can't help but think that a fair number of them would have started earlier if they even suspected there would be a problem. In my experience, for every young woman who is petrified she will have trouble conceiving, there is another who sails through her twenties and thirties convinced "it will happen when it happens."

If I had had my way, and we did wait until "someday" to get pregnant, I can pretty much guarantee you that the "someday" would have turned into "never." With that in mind, here are a few important factors to consider *before* you stall (or, conversely, rush into) having a baby. Some of them you know. Some of them you don't. But *all* of them should at least be taken into account before you cavalierly declare what the "right time" ought to be.

REASONS TO RUSH:

1. The Biological Clock

I know, you've heard it all before. "My clock is ticking." "My eggs are getting old." "I better have kids before it's too late." Blah, blah, blah. Well, guess what? Her clock is ticking, her eggs are getting old, and she better have kids before it's too late. Now, granted, a woman's tone might be so bitter and so vindictive when she says these things that you'd think the entire male gender had actually *planned* it that way—but it still doesn't make her dreaded "clock" any less real.

For those of you who spaced out during 10th-grade biology, let me give you a quick refresher course. Unlike men, who are constantly producing new sperm, a woman is born with a lifetime supply of eggs—and as she ages, so does that supply of precious genetic material. In fact, studies have shown that a woman's eggs start to degenerate by the ripe young age of 27. Twenty-seven! Hell, when I was 27, my mom was still doing my laundry!

Now, here's the even more shocking part. Most women are completely unaware of this fact (lucky for you, I guess). Go ahead, ask them. Even ask the ones who gave you the death look when they talked about the dreaded biological clock. They'll tell you it starts to tick louder at 30, 35, even 40. And they're not just saying it to "trick" you into a false sense of security either. They honestly, truly believe it. This is the myth perpetuated by a society fixated on youth and career—not to mention the countless celebrities singing the praises of childbirth after 40. (Nearly all of them through donor eggs, I assure you.)

In 2001 the American Society for Reproductive Medicine ran a series of subway and bus ads in New York City. The picture in the ad showed an hourglass-shaped baby bottle with a caption that read, "*Advanced Age Decreases Your Ability to Have Children.*" Sadly the campaign was quickly scrapped because of too many complaints—most of them from women's organizations who deemed the whole thing sexist. I often wonder how many childless 41-year-olds could have avoided that fertility office waiting room if only they'd had a chance to read those ads.

The biological clock is real, guys. And not only when it comes to getting pregnant. The longer a woman waits, the greater her risk for miscarriage, premature deliveries, birth defects, and complications during pregnancy. Just think of your wife as Michael Jordan when he retired at 36. (Only shorter and with a much weaker jump shot.) Michael certainly wasn't "old," at least by life span standards, but even he knew that his ability to fly through the air had certainly diminished with age. Now imagine M.J. taking that same basketball, carrying it in his stomach for nine months, and then pushing it out through his asshole. You get the picture.

2. Medical History

My wife has ulcerative colitis. For those of you who don't know what that is, you don't want to. Put (mercifully) simply she has ulcers all up and down her colon, and, because of it, she's been known to shit as much as 20 times a day. See? I told you you didn't want to know. But the point is, this was a preexisting condition that, despite many experts stating otherwise, might very well have contributed to her inability to get pregnant. (By the way, we never did find out why we couldn't get pregnant. "Unexplained infertility" is all we were ever told—a diagnosis that is as frustrating as it is common.[1])

So if you, your wife, or any of your immediate family members have or have had any physical or medical conditions that you even suspect might make it harder to get pregnant, don't shrug it off. And I'm not just talking the obvious stuff. Things as seemingly insignificant as your wife never getting pregnant during her wild college days, or you trying hard to block out that most painful and embarrassing paintball injury (seriously, I know the guy) could very well point to fertility problems.

---

[1]According to a recent study by the Practice Committee of the American Society for Reproductive Medicine, roughly 15–30 percent of all infertility cases are unexplained. In other words, no direct cause can be found in either partner despite often extensive testing.

I recommend you and your wife take a few minutes to discuss your families' medical histories and potential trouble spots. Were there any relatives who had difficulty conceiving? Do you recall hearing about a lot of miscarriages? Was your boyhood home next to a nuclear power plant? (Yes, I know that guy, too.) There's no way of saying what will or won't prove significant, but, in the end, the more you know about your past, the more control you'll ultimately have over your future.

DR. ROSEN: One quick thing to add here. While there are many medical conditions that can contribute to infertility, there are almost none that are guaranteed to make you infertile or sterile. So while it's important to consider all possible roadblocks, you shouldn't drive yourself (or your wife) crazy with it. Case in point: I once treated a woman who was so obsessed with discovering the hidden root of her infertility, she completely overlooked the simple fact that she forgot to remove her IUD.

3. Gut Feeling

I'm a pragmatist. I don't put much stock in fate or luck or destiny for most anything. But when it comes to "gut feelings," especially in the fertility world, I gotta pay some heed.

My wife always said that she'd have trouble conceiving. Right from the very first time we discussed it. She had no real evidence to support this—except maybe the fact that she'd never been pregnant before, and she suffered from the afore-mentioned ulcerative colitis—but she still "felt" strongly that there would be a problem.

Now, as far as I can see, two things may account for the fact that she was right: (1) people are more in tune with their physiology than we give them credit for, or (2) the fear of having fertil-ity problems brought on enough stress to cause fertility problems. In other words, it was a self-fulfilling prophecy.

Whatever the reason, the fact remains. She said she would have trouble conceiving, and she did. If your wife is the same way, then don't ignore it. Believe me, no woman wants to come out and tell her husband that she fears she won't conceive. This is sacred ground for women, and your wife wouldn't dare bring it up if she didn't seriously think it was true. It would be like a man warning his wife that he'll probably be impotent some day.

Could she just be saying this to trick you into having kids before you're ready? Maybe. But now we're getting into issues of trust and deception that are really for another book. I think Dr. Phil wrote a good one on the subject if you're interested.

REASONS TO STALL

1. Financial Considerations

If you haven't said these words before, then you at least know someone who has. "We can't have a baby yet. We can't afford it." And maybe it's true. According to the USDA, the average cost for raising a child is about $15,000 a year.

But here's the deal, guys. As much as that kid costs to raise, it's nothing compared to the cost of infertility treatments, let alone any complications that might arise from a high-risk pregnancy. Around the time of our fifth IVF, I remember my wife and I used to joke, "You mean there are people out there who can just have sex and get pregnant for free?" With any luck, you're still young enough to be one of those people, and, believe me, it's nothing to take for granted.

And one more thing: Having met enough reluctant fathers in my day (and I put myself at the top of that list), I know how strong the desire can be to find any reason—and money's always a great one—for putting off having that kid as long as possible. Just don't fall into the trap of confusing financial prudence with a run-of-the-mill excuse. As I said before, depending on your circumstances, having kids now could be the deal of the century!

2. Lifestyle changes

I ain't gonna lie to you. Having a baby is not an easy gig. And chances are it will affect every aspect of your life—from your work, to your free time, to your sleep schedule (*especially* your sleep schedule). If all, or any, of that doesn't sit well with you right now, then this is the time to bring it up. If your reasons are valid, and have a foreseeable end in sight, then it might be wise to wait a while. If, however, your reasons are decidedly lame, or if you can't commit to a firm start date, then you might want to think about what's *really* holding you back. Remember all those pathetic excuses you gave her about why you couldn't get married yet? It's kind of like that.[2]

So before you go jumping headlong into the fabulous world of unprotected "baby" sex, it might not hurt to consider the timing just a little bit. Are you months away from completing an educational or training program? Did you just start a new job? Are you on the road a lot? These are just a few of the many reasons you might want to *legitimately* hold off on having kids for a little while.

Now, I say "legitimately" because, as with financial considerations, you don't want to fall into the trap of hollow excuses ("as soon as I get that promotion" being a good example).

3. Desire for kids

Throughout our fertility nightmare—damn it, there I go again!—I mean, fertility process, I always used to say, "I *want* kids. My wife *needs* kids." She needed them bad. Like air and water. And, needless to say, this played a very important

---

[2]For the record: My argument for putting off having children was that we'd no longer be able to go out for dinner seven nights a week. Needless to say, it didn't fly.

part in what we did, when we did it, and how many sacrifices we were willing to make along the way.

Not everyone has the same goals and the same dreams, and it's important—no, it's vital— that you and your wife sit down and discuss how "urgent" a priority having children will be. Start with the basics. Do you even want kids? You'd be amazed how many men would secretly prefer to live a life of coupled bliss, and if that's you, now's the time to say it. Believe me, the truth will come out eventually, and it's better to get it out on the table now than after you've spent much of your time, energy, and savings on fertility treatments.

Will having this conversation with your wife be easy? Of course not. Chances are it will be awkward and uncomfortable, just like most everything else in the fertility world. (Wait until I get to procreation sex in the next chapter.) To make matters worse, it might even fall upon you to initiate the discussion. You see, assuming there *are* fertility concerns, your wife is very scared right now. I know she might not say it, and, instead, she might take it out on you by being short-tempered or extra emotional, but believe me, she is scared. And the last thing she wants to do is scare herself even more by finding out that her husband may not even want to have children at all. So take a deep breath, find a good time, and have this awkward talk.

And if she resists, tell her that she made you read this stupid book in the first place, so now she damn well better listen to what it says.

So what's the bottom line? If your wife is under 30, you're both healthy, and there are no obvious indications of fertility issues, then don't sweat it. Frankly, I'm more concerned about why you're reading this book in the first place!

If, on the other hand, your wife is over 30 *and* has reason to suspect a fertility problem, then definitely give yourself at least one more year to have children than you otherwise would. Keep in mind that a year is nothing in the fertility world. Between waiting on menstrual cycles (sorry, gross word), dealing with potential setbacks, and replenishing funds, a year or two can come and go in a heartbeat. And as far as I'm concerned, it's still better to find yourself unprepared for fatherhood than to never be a father at all.

So what the heck are you waiting for?! Start trying. Now. Put the book down and go. I mean it. Why are you still reading? Stop it. The clock is ticking. Tick, tick, tick, tick tick . . .

2

WHEN TO TRY HARDER

You probably won't even notice at first, but at some point after you guys have been "trying" for a while—maybe three to six months into it—your wife will start acting a bit strangely. She'll stare longingly at passing babies in the mall. She'll look for any excuse to talk about infants, pregnancy, baby clothes, birth, parenthood, or preschools. She'll view sex as more of a "means to an end" than a pleasurable activity—and, chances are, it's this last one that will clue you in to something being terribly, terribly wrong here.

In fact, what's wrong is that you guys may have trouble conceiving, and, like most everything else in your life, your wife picked up on it long before you did. Want proof? Go check the medicine cabinet. Alongside the home pregnancy tests that you may or may not have known were there, you'll probably find a couple of ovulation predictor kits and an extra thermometer. What's all that shit for, you may ask? Well, I'm gonna tell you.

- **Taking temperature.** Here's another one I bet you didn't know. When a woman is about to ovulate (in other words, her time to get knocked up), a hormone called progesterone causes her body temperature to dip slightly and then sharply rise. So by taking her temperature at regular, obsessive intervals, she can look out for that spike and, presto, know exactly when to pretend she's really horny. That's the theory, at least. In truth, lots of things other than hormones can affect her body's temperature, so this method of ovulation prediction is shaky at best. All the same, you'd be best served to just let her have her fun and play along. Worst-case scenario, she'll make you have sex for nothing. Boo-hoo.

- **Ovulation prediction kits.** Once your wife has grown tired of the whole thermometer thing, she'll probably turn to ovulation predictor kits. This method of ovulation prediction uses your wife's pee to test for hormone levels, so you gotta figure it's more accurate than mere temperature alone.[3] Still not 100 percent accurate, but, again,

---

[3]*DR. ROSEN: The hormone in the urine is called LH (short for luteinizing hormone), and it is only present for about 24 to 36 hours prior to ovulation. A positive result means that the woman will ovulate in the next one to three days (with an 85 percent accuracy rate).*

if it makes her feel like she has more control over the process, then I say don't mess with it. Just don't let her use them six at a time like my wife did. As hard as this was for her to accept, they're all gonna read the same thing.

- **Saliva tests.** Yet another over-the-counter predictor, except this one uses spit rather than pee. (Delightful, isn't it?) The good news is that saliva tests are at least as accurate as the other tests mentioned. The bad news is they can cost as much as 60 bucks a pop (as opposed to 15 bucks for the pee variety). So unless you got an extra 45 bucks to . . . well . . . *piss* away, then I say stick to the cheaper ones.

- **Charting the results.** A lot of this prediction business, particularly the thermometer stuff, requires keeping accurate charts and/or graphs of your temperature at any given point. Thankfully my wife is as unorganized as I am, so I was merely subjected to a few scraps of paper with numbers on them. Some women, however—your computer whizzes, scrapbookers and list makers in particular—will be brandishing their Excel spreadsheets and/or returning from Staples with posterboard, Sharpies, mounting tape, and a ruler. Again, it's all about her feeling in control, so just go with it. The last thing you want to do is make your wife feel stupid, ashamed, or secretive about any of this.

Procreation Sex

Remember in junior high when you thought there was no such thing as bad sex? It could have been with the lunch lady, your friend's grandmother, a halfway-decent-looking leper. Didn't matter. Just so long as you'd be getting some. Well that was long before you heard about a little thing called "procreation sex." In other words, the planned, mandatory acts of copulation that will be required as your wife charts her monthly cycle.

It's a fascinating thing, this procreation sex. When you really come down to it, procreation is the only reason sex exists in the first place. And yet for most guys (myself included), the thought of doing it solely for the purpose of childbearing is about as sexy as watching water buffalos going at it on *Animal Planet*. For one thing, there's absolutely no spontaneity. You're pretty much going to know a day in advance that you *will* be having sex tomorrow. Not might be. *Will* be. And don't think she's gonna say it in some sweet, seductive tone of voice, either. No, it's gonna sound pretty much like when she asks you to take out the garbage for the umpteenth time. But even more persistent and bossy. Like it's really smelly garbage that already has rats and raccoons poking at it.

It's not that she's mean, and it's not that she's insensitive. (Unless, of course, your wife is already mean and insensitive, in which case I can't help you.) It's just that she wants to have a baby really, really bad, and sex still happens to be the most convenient way for that to happen. Women can do that, you know. They can have sex for different reasons. Sometimes for love, sometimes for sport, sometimes for security, sometimes for babies.

So how do you give in to her lousy procreation sex demands without feeling like some sort of indentured sperm donor? Here's a few thoughts:

1. Tell her to chill

There's a fine line between aggressor and tyrant, and a woman hungry for procreation sex tends to cross it a lot. If this bothers you (as it did me), let her know. Calmly explain that you don't so much mind being told when you're going to have sex as you do being told 30 times. She just has to say it once. You won't forget. You'll be there with bells on (if that's your thing). At least this way you can *pretend* that you had something to do with it in the first place.

2. Tell her not to lie to you

Now that you've made her so self-conscious about the whole procreation sex thing, she'll probably avoid the subject altogether the next time and opt instead for the old "I'm so horny tonight" routine. Do they think we're that dumb? Apparently my wife did for more than a year, and I really didn't like it. It made me feel cheap. Like that girl in college who I said I loved just so I could sleep with her. I'd apologize to her now, but for the life of me I can't remember her name.

3. Seize the opportunity to spice things up

Never, at any time in your marriage, will you have a sweeter opportunity to say "Okay, fine. But as long as we have to do it, why not try that *thing* we once talked about?" Any fetish. Any fantasy. You name it. You are in such a great bargaining position here, it's not even funny! And besides, it's not like your kid's ever gonna know that he was conceived with

Daddy tied to the bed and Mommy in a dominatrix outfit, right?

4. Don't limit yourself to once a month

Just because you're forced to have sex a couple of days a month, doesn't mean all the other days have to be ruined. In fact, I encourage you to have good old-fashioned recreational sex as often as you can when you know you *can't* get pregnant. This will help take the edge off the dreaded "procreation sex" at mid-cycle.

DR. ROSEN: Believe it or not, there is even data to suggest that if a guy abstains for more than two or three days, the couple's chance of conceiving actually decreases. Yet another reason not to "save up" for the dreaded day.

3

WHEN TO WORRY

So your wife just turned 35, you've been trying for six months, and all you've got to show for it is a drugstore's worth of negative pregnancy tests. Is this really bad? Is it time to see a doctor? I'll give you the answer that I heard most often when I was going through this. It's the same answer I got when I was shopping for a house, choosing the right puppy and, yes, even deciding when to get married:

"You'll just know."

I realize that sounds kind of pat. At least that's what I thought when I heard it. But it's still no less true. There will come a day—maybe after three months, maybe after three years—when both you and your wife know, in your heart of hearts, that something is truly amiss. That's the easy part. The hard part is actually doing something about it. Especially if your wife is reluctant to admit there's a problem.

DR. ROSEN: As a general rule, no woman of child-bearing age should need more than three to four months to get pregnant. In fact, roughly 85 percent of people who are going to get pregnant in the first year do so within six months. Any longer than this, and it might be time to consider a specialist.

Doers vs. Avoiders

While there's no telling how your wife will react to the sobering prospect of infertility, I can pretty much guarantee that she will fall into one of two very distinct categories—the Doers and the Avoiders—that roughly break down like this:

> **The Doers:** These are the women who, as soon as they suspect there's a problem, shift into high gear and make things happen. Books will be bought, lectures will be attended, appointments will be made. The Doers don't waste time, and they don't take shit from nobody. My wife was a Doer. She was the ultimate Doer. She was a tornado.

> **The Avoiders:** These are the women who believe that, so long as they don't acknowledge there's a problem, they don't have a problem. They become detached, closed off, emotionless. In other words, very much like men.[4]

---

[4]While many of you, in the short run, may appreciate a wife who's this adept at sweeping such an unpleasant subject under the rug, in the long run it might wind up causing more problems than it solves.

Oddly enough, there's no telling which one of these classifications your wife will fall into until she's forced to make a choice. I've seen the most powerful, domineering women practically crawl into a shell when faced with fertility problems and, conversely, I've seen the most shy, passive women suddenly able to take on the world. Furthermore, there's no telling if, and when, an Avoider will become a Doer and vice versa. It all comes down to how much they can take at any given point.

Here's the bottom line: If you've honestly reached that point where you *know* there's a problem, and your wife isn't doing enough about it, then it is your duty and your obligation to pick up the slack. Fertility problems do not go away. They only get worse. With that being said, here are some simple, straightforward ways for you to take control of the situation and make things happen:

Communicate

It's the most important thing you can do. It's always the most important thing. Ask your wife if she's concerned about going this long without getting pregnant. Does she think there might be a problem? Should you guys maybe take some action? The key here is to be as casual and nonconfrontational as possible. My advice is to play dumb. It always works for me! In other words, you're not *telling* her there's a problem. You're *asking* her—since she's so much smarter than you with these sorts of things—if she *thinks* there might be one.

A fair warning: You are about to broach a subject that cuts to the very core of what it means to be a woman (at least as far as most wives are concerned). This is like trying to tap into a 50,000-watt electrical tower without shutting down the power first. One wrong move, and you're fried. However, if timed right and handled correctly, you will score some *major* brownie points for your extreme caring and concern.

Educate

Let's assume you had the talk, and, despite your wife's admitting there's a problem, she still won't take any action. Now it's time to start educating both of you on what your options might be. Surf the Internet, find a book or two on the subject, watch that biweekly "infertility" episode of Dr. Oz.

Remember, you can't just rely solely on your wife for information. Sometimes you've got to take the bull by the horns and find things out for yourself.

Support

Many women choose to go at this whole process alone. My wife was one of those. Due partly to denial, and partly to embarrassment, she decided that it was best to handle this without the support of friends, family, or any outside organizations. In fact, when I suggested we attend an infertility support group, she scoffed at the very notion, claiming that she wasn't one of "those women." I still don't know exactly who "those women" were, but I felt all too certain that she was, in fact, one of them.

In what might be my proudest early moment of this process, I took the brave initiative of contacting an online infertility support group and explaining our situation. At first my wife was uninterested in, even dismissive of, the responses. But as the many posts came in—and as she saw, and felt, the support of so many other women like herself—it was as if a great weight was no longer being carried entirely by herself. There was help out there. And she was finally ready to accept it.

DR. ROSEN: What Marc is describing is really true in a majority of women. They initially want no one to know. A lot of infertile women treat infertility like a drug or drinking problem. They want to hide it from everyone, and the best thing you can do, as her partner in life, is get her to talk about it and help her find out that she is not alone.

A word of warning about the Internet: Like most online topics, the sheer number of infertility-related sites can be daunting, and there's no guarantee that any one you click on is reputable. My advice is to start with www.resolve.com or www.protectyourfertility. com. Here you'll find all the information you need to get going.

The 10 Things Not to Say to Your Fertility-Challenged Wife:

1) That's okay. I didn't want you to get fat anyway.

2) No more condoms? Cool!

3) Can't we just invest all that money in a flat screen instead?

4) Yes, but these doctors have yet to see my Super Sperm!

5) So if your sister carries it, does that mean I can finally sleep with her?

6) I don't even want kids.

7) Hey, did I tell you my ex-girlfriend's pregnant?

8) I discussed it with my mother, and she thinks . . .

9) Don't worry. You're still relatively young.

10) But it's not *my* fault, right?

ROUND TWO
SPRING TRAINING

This is it, guys. You've spent months, maybe even years, trying to convince yourself that it's only a matter of time before you get pregnant, and suddenly you realize that time may very well be running out. That's not a bad thing, though. In fact, it's a good thing. Congratulations. Because now you're finally ready to embark on the most important, and often most dreaded, step of your infertility journey: seeing the doctor.

In this section we'll talk about what you should expect from a good fertility doctor, what he should expect from you, and how to best prepare yourself for the startling changes that are about to take place—in your wife, in your marriage, and in your overall perception of what it means to "get pregnant."

4

THE FERTILITY DOCTOR

Okay, so you've been trying for a while, you've done the research, you've gotten the support, and still no baby. There's no more fighting it. It's time to seek out a professional. For many people, this will start with a visit to their family doctor. For others, like myself (actually, like my wife; I just tagged along), we cut right to the chase and went to directly to a fertility specialist. Either way, you should both be congratulated for taking the initiative and confronting this potentially serious problem head-on.

Now, before we get into what *you* can expect from this encounter, let's just take a moment to look at it from your wife's point of view. As I said before, your wife's ability to conceive cuts to the very core of what it means to be a woman, and more than likely she is feeling scared, ashamed, depressed, embarrassed, and inadequate. Some women will admit to these feelings. Others will not. It's up to you to assume the feelings are there and act accordingly. Be considerate, be patient, be supportive. In other words, from the moment you enter that office till the moment you leave, be a man.

That's it, lecture over. Now let's get back to how all this affects *you*.

The Invisible Man

Ever wonder why infertility books aren't written for men? Simple. Because nobody gives a shit about the man! Just take one look at a fertility clinic's waiting room, and you'll know what I'm talking about. Chances are it's done up in flowery pastels. The men's bathroom, if there is one, is often at the other end of the building and requires a key with a giant shoehorn on the end for entry. And the closest thing to a guys' magazine you're gonna find is a copy of *American Baby* with a scantily clad Denise Richards on the cover.

At first this bothered me. A lot. I mean, as an equal partner in this process, don't I play just as vital a role in its ultimate success or failure? In a word: no. In 10 words: Positively not at all in any way, shape, or form. Like pregnancy itself, the woman carries most of the burden when it comes to infertility. She takes the shots, she gets the procedures (most of them, at least), she feels the pain. So it only makes sense that she should get most of the attention as well. Just be thankful for it and shut up. To give you an idea of what I'm talking about, the chart that follows contains a partial list of all the procedures my wife and I went through during our six-year odyssey, along with each of our respective roles throughout. As you'll see, most, in fact nearly all, of these tests revolve around the woman, whereas the man's role—if there even is one—comes down to just one word. Sperm. Give 'em a little of that and your testing is pretty much over. It rarely gets more complicated than that.

At the risk of objectifying your wife, you can almost think of her as a luxury automobile going in for a full inspection to diagnose a problem. They have to get under the hood, check the engine, tests the fluids, make sure all the hoses are working properly . . . and when all is said and done, you just need to pump a little gas in the tank.

Oh, and one quick word of warning: Turn this page at your own risk. What follows may contain details that will throw your wife into an unrecoverable tailspin. And rest assured that *very* few people subject themselves to this much torture. As I said before, my wife is the Doer's Doer.

Procedure	Her Role	My Role
Internal Ultrasound	Spread her legs in stirrups while a male doctor and his male assistant shoved a "giant dildo" (her words) inside her and "fished around."	Nothing.
Clomid Pills	Used to increase egg production, they left her body bloated and her face broken out. Other side effects include depression and hot flashes.	Nothing.
(16) Artificial Inseminations	Spread legs in the trusty stirrups while a nurse injected my sperm directly into her cervix through a soft catheter	Jerked off in cup.
Gonadotropin shots	Also for egg production, these painful injections left her hormonally imbalanced, bloated, and broken out.	Nothing.
HSG Test	An extremely painful procedure that requires shooting dye directly into the uterus and analyzing the results via X-ray.	Nothing.
Untold number of blood tests	Permanent scar tissue on veins.	Nothing.[5]
(10) In Vitro Fertilizations	Received a seemingly unending number of painful	Jerked off in cup.

(continued)

Procedure	Her Role	My Role
	injections that resulted in severe pain, bloating, and irritability. Also, surgery to remove as many as 27 eggs from her ovaries, which were then combined with my sperm and reimplanted back into her uterus a few days later as embryos.	
G.I.F.T.	Similar to IVF, except in this case the unfertilized eggs and sperm are implanted directly into the fallopian tubes via three arthroscopic-type holes in the belly.	Jerked off in cup.
Laparoscopic or Hysteroscopic Myomectomy	Fibroids are surgically removed from the uterus to make embryo transfer easier and improve chance of pregnancy.	Nothing.
Manual Dilation	A barbaric procedure that involved twisting increasingly larger metal probes into her cervix with the goal of stretching it out to make the embryo transfer easier. Unimaginable pain.	Nothing.

---

⁵ That's actually not true. I was asked to take a blood test around our fifth IVF, and passed out from light-headedness.

Given this obvious disparity, a husband's first instinct might be to step back and let his wife handle everything. I mean, clearly he doesn't have that much to offer, right? Well, physically, no. But emotionally and psychologically, a husband's input can be immeasurably important—especially at the beginning of this process when his wife's emotions, uncertainties, and insecurities are probably at their height.

So with that in mind, here are some helpful ways to make your presence known at those initial consultations, even if the fertility doctor doesn't so much as look at you.

1. Prepare questions

Come on, I know you have at least a few. You don't? Okay, well then here are some easy ones to get you going: "What factors make one doctor's success rate higher than another?" "Are there any procedures you don't endorse?" "Why do you think infertility has become so prevalent?" "Could you tell us a little about your background?"

As you can see, the questions you ask at an initial consultation need not require any technical knowledge or prior research. I think a lot of people get intimidated by entering into a field they know very little about. I know I did. The truth of the matter is, picking your fertility doctor, at its most basic level, is no different from picking your plumber or electrician. You're looking for a guy (or gal) who seems knowledgeable, trustworthy, comes highly recommended and, perhaps most important, is *someone you can get along with.* Remember, this person will be privy to your most intimate feelings and private moments. If you, in any way, feel uncomfortable around him or her, then move on to someone else. Believe me, there's another doctor just as good who you *can* get along with.

2. Listen

Sounds easy, right? But you'd be amazed how much of the information you'll hear will go in one ear and out the other. Remember, your mind is going to be reeling at this point (and your wife's twice as much). You'll be bombarded with all sorts of facts, statistics, and *COSTS.* The more you can stay focused in the present, the better off you'll be. You might even want to take notes. Not only will this help you to retain all the information, but it will help score some *major* brownie points with the overwhelmed wife. (Again, the most important thing when all is said and done.)

3. Go to *every* consultation you can

I mean it, guys. You can't claim to be involved if you don't even show up for the initial consultations. As you'll quickly discover, every doctor is different—maybe not in the technology they're using, but certainly in their outlooks, their attitudes, their opinions. Having your wife just relay this information to you when you get home isn't nearly enough. You really have to be there. For solidarity's sake, if nothing else.

4. Bring your own reading material

I wasn't kidding when I talked about the magazines in the waiting room. You're going to be hard pressed to find anything that doesn't have a baby, a pregnant woman, or Sarah Jessica Parker on the cover. You're also, more than likely, going to be sitting in that pastel prison a hell of a lot longer than you will with the doctor, so be sure to bring your own reading material (or work, or Nintendo DS, etc.) to keep yourself busy. Not only will this make the experience easier for you, but there's only so many "when's he gonna see us already's" your nervous wife can take.

5. Respect the office staff

These are the people who *really* make the office run. They schedule your appointments; they deal with your insurance company; they administer, or assist with, virtually all of the procedures. So if you go into this thing treating them like the waitress who forgot your hot wings at Hooters, you're gonna be setting yourself (and your wife) up for one hell of a nasty ride. Whether it's in your nature or not, you gotta come off like the sweetest, most good-natured, metrosexual partner who ever stepped foot in their office. I'm telling you—they love that guy! Now this isn't to say you shouldn't turn into Mr. Asshole if the situation warrants it, but that attitude, or anything close to it, should truly be your last resort.

One final thing to keep in mind when choosing a doctor. Proximity. It may not seem like such a big deal now to drive 20 miles for an appointment, but as more treatments are required, so are more visits. An IVF treatment, for example, might require a trip to the doctor nearly every day. And you can pretty much kiss goodbye bringing in any semen samples from home as they, like Domino's Pizza, must be delivered in under 30 minutes. (See chapter 9 for more on this lovely subject.)

DR. ROSEN: I'd like to second everything Marc said, and add a few points of my own. First off, choosing the right doctor is huge (and I'm not just saying that because I am one). The family doctor that you've been going to since you got your first booster shots at age four is probably not the best choice. A general ob-gyn may be a good place to start for your evaluation, but ideally he or she should be a reproductive endocrinologist as well. These subspecialists have spent an extra two or three years in training to deal specifically with infertility cases. If, however, you require in vitro fertilization (discussed more in chapter 10), you will need to see a board-certified reproductive endocrinologist, as opposed to someone merely trained in that procedure.

So how do you choose the right doctor for you? Well, by and large, there are three criteria that should come into play: (1) How well does he treat you as a couple and address your concerns, (2) How well does he answer your questions, and (3) Will he develop a diagnostic and treatment plan that is individual for you? When you call for the initial consultation, be sure to ask how much time the doctor plans to spend with you. If the answer is 45 minutes or more, then all your concerns will probably be addressed. If, on the other hand, he plans on pawning you off to his ancillary staff after 10–20 minutes, then you might want to look elsewhere.

MARC: Besides a list of questions, is there anything else new patients should bring with them for this initial consultation?

DR. ROSEN: Yes, any medical records from any prior testing or treatment.

MARC: And, typically, what would you cover in this first meeting?

DR. ROSEN: After reviewing the couple's history and answering all their questions, I usually lay out a plan for their fertility problem, explain all the tests as well as the ramifications of normal vs. abnormal results, what the time frame is for these tests, their cost, and when we will be talking again. I typically won't examine a woman during the initial visit (though 10–20 percent of the time I will) and I never examine the men. At least not yet. We'll save all those pleasantries for the next section.

MARC: I can't wait!

5

"WHO *ARE* YOU?"

Before getting married I was the most reluctant of all reluctant grooms. I basically equated marriage with death. Can't explain why. Still don't know, in fact. All I can say is that for about a year or so leading up to my wedding, I was pretty much a basket case.

During this (sorry, honey) awful time in my life, I remember very clearly lying in my bed at night with my then fiancée by my side. And in between bouts of cold sweats and intricate plots to run away to foreign countries, I would turn to this beautiful sleeping angel by my side and say out loud, "Who *are* you?" It wasn't that I didn't know her. Or even love her (a lot, for that matter). It was just so weird to look at this person I'd known for less than two years and come to grips with the fact that she was my soul mate for eternity.

Does that make any sense? Probably not. In case you haven't noticed, I'm a little weird. But the point is this: Whether or not you get what I'm talking about now, you sure as hell will when you're going through fertility treatments. Because one way or another, your wife *will* change. Some of the changes will be subtle—like she'll be a bit more sensitive around kids. Other changes will be more significant—like she'll lose that spark that made you fall in love with her in the first place. But regardless of the extent, I guarantee you that at some point in your fertility journey, you're gonna look at that sleeping angel beside you and ponder the same question: "Who are you?"

In nearly all cases, the answer will be as simple as it is complicated: Who is she? She's a mother without children, that's who she is. And until you understand the magnitude of what that means—and how that feels—you'll never be a true partner in this struggle.

As I said before, men want kids. Women *need* them. And when this most basic of needs is ignored, bad shit can result.

Getting Inside Your Wife's Head (Not As Scary As It Sounds)

While no two women will react to infertility in exactly the same way, there are a few universal "truths" that, at least in my experience, seem to apply to all sufferers. Listen closely, guys. These are the pearls. If I could tattoo them on your arm, I would.

UNIVERSAL TRUTH #1:
Fertility-Challenged Women Hate Kids

Sounds completely contradictory, doesn't it? But it's true. By and large, women struggling to have kids will do everything in their power to avoid being around them. It's just too painful. Too much of a reminder of what they don't have. In my own case, this became a real problem after a while. We had to avoid family movies and TV shows. We drifted apart from close friends with children. I even made the difficult choice to not invite one of my wife's best buddies to her surprise 35th birthday party because his wife was six months pregnant at the time (sorry, Gary). That's how overwhelming this aversion had become. Just be conscious and considerate as your wife starts to fall prey to it, and do whatever you can (within reason) to respect its limitations.

UNIVERSAL TRUTH #2:
Fertility-Challenged Women Hate
When People Talk About Their
Fertility-challenged . . . Ness

Again you're thinking, What the hell? Haven't I been stressing communication this entire time? Yes, I have. Communication with *you*. Not your friends. Not your relatives. And especially not your poor grandchild-deprived mother. So along with being supportive and understanding, your job description must also now include running interference every once in a while. I wouldn't go so far as to tell your friends to "shut the hell up" whenever they ask your wife how it's going, but a quiet aside after the fact would certainly go a long way to making her more comfortable and secure.

UNIVERSAL TRUTH #3: Fertility-Challenged Women Hate to be Compared to Other Fertility-Challenged Women (or Non-fertility-Challenged Women, for that Matter)

Now, this isn't to say that they themselves won't constantly compare themselves to other women. They will. Ad nauseam, in fact. It's only when you (or anyone else for that matter) make the comparison that they turn into Linda Blair from *The Exorcist*. Think of it this way: How would you like it if you kept getting passed over for the same promotion at work and, in order to make you feel better, your wife kept telling you about all the other husbands who had absolutely no trouble whatsoever getting promoted? I can remember my mother (who, by the way, has a fantastic relationship with my wife) constantly telling us how easy it was for her to get pregnant with me and my sister—as if somehow this ability would magically transfer to my wife through some sort of fertility osmosis. Similarly, don't think the success stories—you know, women just like her who persevered—will go over any better. If anything, they'll only elicit a "why them and not me?" reaction. And the failures? Hoping that maybe she'll appreciate the "misery loves company" aspect? Nice try, genius. But that one's just gonna make her cry. In the end, when it comes to comparisons, your best bet is just to shut up and let her do all the talking. You know . . . like the old days.

Remember those truths. Memorize them. And be sure not to mess with them as you stumble forward on the bumpy road ahead.

6

STARTING TREATMENT

There's no more denying it. With that first visit to the doctor's office, you and your wife have officially joined the ranks of fellow "infertility sufferers." For some, this label will only be applied for a short time. A few hits of Clomid, and, boom, the little lady's knocked up in no time. For others, the label will stick for what seems like an eternity. However, regardless of what happens from here on out, it's important to remember some words of wisdom we heard at one of our many support groups:

You and your wife will become parents. It might not be now, and it might not be in the way you intended, but one way or another, if your resolve is strong enough, it will happen.

In the next few chapters, we'll look at the many different ways that modern science can help you realize that dream, as well as prepare you for what lies on the road ahead. As I said before, none of this will be easy, but there are certainly a great number of ways to soften the blow.

And just to make it easier for you, I've assigned a "Wife Psycho Level" (ranked from 1 to 10) to each new stage of the process. Here's how the numbers will break down:

"Wife Psycho Level"

1–3: She's stressing a bit, but nothing you can't handle. A couple of nice gestures and a supportive ear, and you'll probably be able to calm her down in no time.

4–6: Her stress level has reached a point where it's starting to affect your marriage and day-to-day lives. She'll act irrationally at times, and your ability to calm her will severely diminish. At this point you might start to wonder who the crazy lady is.

7–9: She is a basket case. Emotionally, physically, and psychologically. Her every waking moment will revolve around infertility, and you'll start to see a totally different person from the one you married. Your ability to soothe her will be nearly nonexistent, and the best you can hope for at this point is to stay clear of her line of fire. These are the critical days and weeks that can make or break your marriage.

10: I'd like to think I never saw 10, that any guy in his right mind would have packed up and left by 10. Ten are those crazy ladies who steal babies from Chuck E. Cheese.

So without further ado, let's dive into this stuff. And what better place to start than with you and your wife as human guinea pigs.

Tests and More Tests (Wife Psycho Level: 3)

After finding a doctor you both feel comfortable with, the next step will be to determine why you guys can't get pregnant. This will require a series of tests ranging from simple blood work to a slew of more complicated and invasive procedures that are almost as hard to pronounce as they are to understand. Whether you guys have some or all of these tests will depend on a great number of factors, ranging from your age to your genetic history to any preexisting conditions that you may or may not already know about. In other words, don't go into this assuming you're getting everything listed below, but, by the same token, don't immediately rule out any of these tests should your doctor suggest them. Remember that the key to solving your infertility problem is knowing what the problem is in the first place—so the sooner you guys can find that out, the better.

Now, as you might have already guessed, nearly all of these tests will be performed on your wife, not you (breathe a sigh of relief and silently cheer), but, as I stressed back in chapter 3, that isn't your cue to just check out or, worse yet, gloat about it when you get back home. As with all phases of this process, it's important to stay somewhat involved with what she's doing or, at the very least, create the *illusion* that you are. So, with that in mind, here's a quick cheat sheet of what may or may not lie ahead for the mother of your children-to-be. And rest assured, this is as technical as I'll ever get.

DR. ROSEN: I won't let you off that easy. So if long, acronymed medical jargon tends to give you headaches, I suggest you skip this chapter altogether (though I sincerely wish you wouldn't).

I'd also like to point out that the majority of these tests should be completed within the first two to three months, and, pending the results, any follow-up treatment should commence soon thereafter.

 ## BLOOD TESTS:

Marc's Cheat Sheet

Summary: Tests various levels of stuff related to fertility. Abnormal levels may result in further testing or prescribed medication.

Degree of pain: It's a blood test. You figure it out.

What they're testing for: Progesterone level, estradiol level, LH level, FSH level. You'll hear your wife and her friends throwing these numbers around like they're the player stats of a rotisserie baseball league.

Easy brownie points: FSH level should be less than 10, so if she says it's lower, look happy. If she says it's higher, express immediate concern.

Dr. Rosen's Expanded Boring Science Content:

Okay, let's break this down a bit further so you can see what we're really testing for.

FSH is a hormone that the brain releases to get an egg to ripen in the ovary. It is usually measured on the second or third day of a woman's period, when she's still bleeding. The higher the FSH level, the fewer the eggs that are left in the ovary. Remember that a woman is born with a set number of eggs, and when the FSH is elevated, that means that she is getting a little low on the supply; it becomes a lot harder to get pregnant and the chance of miscarriage is higher. Also, when the FSH is high, all those fertility medications stop working. FSH has to be checked simultaneously with another hormone, estradiol. If they aren't drawn together, you won't be able *to decipher if a low FSH is really low or not. For example, Marc correctly pointed out that an FSH level should be <10, but this assumes that the estradiol is also <50.*

Progesterone is the hormone that the ovaries secrete after ovulation. It is required to prepare the uterus for the hoped-for pregnancy and to allow it to grow once the pregnancy attaches to the uterus. As with FSH, progesterone has to be measured at a certain time of the "month" or it is of no value. The best time to measure it is about one week before the period starts. A level of >10 is normally good, unless the patient is on Clomid (more about this drug later), in which case I prefer to see a level >15. Once a baby is growing, the uterus requires even more progesterone, so in early pregnancy a level of >20 is still considered normal.

 ## HYSTEROSALPINGOGRAM (HSG):

Marc's Cheat Sheet:

> **Summary**: An X-ray test that checks for abnormalities in all them-there lady parts.
>
> **Degree of pain**: Don't let this one fool you. Because of the dye that's injected to see better, this test can be extremely uncomfortable—especially if there are blockages that require that dye to be pushed more forcefully.

What they're testing for: Anything that can block or disrupt the normal flow of things or irritate the uterus.

Easy brownie points: If she mentions a pending "HSG Test," nod sympathetically and say you've heard it can cause some cramping. Then ask if there's anything you can do to help, which, of course, there won't be.

Dr. Rosen's Expanded Boring Science Content:

During an HSG (don't even try to pronounce the full name), a clear liquid that looks white on an X-ray is injected into the interior of the uterus (where the embryo is going to attach). It will then flow out the tubes and spill into the belly. The purpose is to see if there is something in the uterus that could make it more difficult for the pregnancy to attach. These include fibroids, polyps, and scar tissue:

- *Fibroids (also called myomas) are benign (non-cancerous, for the most part) muscle tumors that about a third of all women have. These fibroids can be very small or as big as a cantaloupe. The size of a fibroid is important, but fibroids are like real estate. The location is the primary indicator of their importance. For example, a fibroid on the outside of the uterus, no matter how large, rarely causes a reproductive problem. Conversely, a fibroid near the area where an embryo is suppose to implant, no matter how small, can definitely cause infertility. The good news is that these fibroids can be easily, and relatively painlessly, removed.*

- *Polyps, like fibroids, are primarily benign and resemble small, rounded mushrooms. They are also softer than fibroids, which are typically firm to the touch.*

- *Scar tissue is scar tissue. You only get it from previous surgery inside the uterus or with a few infections.*

All of these entities may cause infertility by irritating the interior of the uterus and allowing less space for a pregnancy to attach and grow. The main reason for this test, however, is to see if the tubes are open. If the tubes are blocked, the egg and sperm can't meet.

 ## HYSTEROSCOPY:

Marc's Cheat Sheet:

Summary: A glorified HSG test to detect smaller polyps and fibroids.

Degree of pain: While this is technically more invasive than your normal HSG (a small tube is inserted directly into the uterus), it is probably less painful thanks to a local anesthetic or mild sedation.

What they're testing for: Same as the HSG, but this procedure can find even smaller polyps, fibroids, and scar tissue that can't be detected with a normal HSG.

Easy brownie points: "Just make sure they numb you for that one!"

Dr. Rosen's Expanded Boring Science Content:

There are two types of hysteroscopy. One is done to diagnose polyps, fibroids, and scar tissue, and the other is to remove these buggers. The latter is usually done in an operating room. What's nice about this procedure is that the recovery is very fast. For example, a woman can have a walnut-size fibroid removed from the inside of her uterus and go to work the next day without any residual pain. One other rule: No sex for at least a few days after an HSG or hysteroscopy.

 ## HUHNER TEST, A.K.A. POSTCOITAL TEST:

Marc's Cheat Sheet:

Summary: Okay, this one does involve you. Around the time of your wife's ovulation, you will be required to have sex with her (yes, I know, it's an awful thing, but somebody's got to do it). The next day the doctor will take a sample of her "stuff" (which now has your stuff, too), and look at it under a microscope.

Degree of pain: I guess that all depends on how well endowed you are.

What they're checking for: The quality and movement of your sperm, as well as the condition of her mucus (believe me, I held off using that word for as long as I could).

Easy brownie points: If you recall from chapter 2, procreation sex can be a bit of a drag. Do whatever you can to make the encounter as exciting and nonclinical as possible.

Dr. Rosen's Expanded Boring Science Content:

Not all doctors do this test, but I think it's a great one to use to determine if intrauterine inseminations might be helpful. Also, a lot of doctors will let you look at the mucus under the microscope, so this test can even become a sort of Discovery Channel event.

After sex, the sperm have to get out of the vagina and into the cervix, which is the entry point into the uterus. Sperm are literally sucked into the cervix and pushed up to the tubes, where the egg should be waiting, so what you should see with a good test are dozens and dozens of sperm swimming in the mucus. A normal test is pretty cool to see, and an abnormal test is pretty easy to understand. A bad test is observed when (1) the sperm are all dead; (2) no sperm, or only a few sperm, are seen swimming along; or (3) the sperm that are present are not moving in a forward manner but are only shaking or quivering in place. (This latter problem is very rare and can be caused by antibodies that some women make to stop sperm. If this is found, a blood test can be done to confirm the result.) If this test is positive, treatment is with IVF. (More about IVF in future chapters.) If this test is done more than two days before or after ovulation, the mucus won't allow sperm to move up into the uterus and either no sperm will be seen or only dead ones. If these findings are observed when the woman is ovulating, these women may benefit from inseminations. (More about those later as well.)

THYROID TESTING:

Marc's Cheat Sheet:

> **What they're checking for**: To see if her thyroid is in balance. If not, it could be a contributing factor to infertility.
>
> **Degree of pain**: Just a blood test.
>
> **Easy brownie points**: If her thyroid is out of whack, stress how great it is that they can regulate it with simple medication.

Dr. Rosen's Expanded Boring Science Content:

Thyroid is a small hormone with a big job: it controls the metabolism—in other words, how the entire body works. For example, women who have too much thyroid hormone (HYPERthyroid) usually have a resting tremor (their hands shake), their heart rate is fast, they lose weight without trying, and they do not tolerate hot weather very well. Women who have too little thyroid hormone (HYPOthyroid) have the opposite problem. They are sleepy, have problems concentrating, they gain weight, and cold weather bothers them. Anyway, it's an easy test, and it's easy to treat.

DR. ROSEN: Marc? (no response) *Marc?*

MARC: What? Oh sorry, I think I fell asleep. Anyway, now that we've highlighted some of the more common tests your wife may or may not be in for, let's move on to the one test that *really* matters—as least as far as us guys are concerned.

The Semen Analysis Test

Allow me to step back in time for a moment. You're 13 years old. For months now, you've been experimenting with the most fantastic new discovery that involves your penis, your mom's Nivea hand cream, and an old issue of *Playboy* that you found in your dad's sock drawer. Discretion is the key here, as you could think of nothing more humiliating than someone actually finding out what you're doing in the bathroom for three hours a day.

Fast-forward 20 years. The Nivea has long since expired, the Playboy is now an old VHS copy of "Hard Dick Drives," but the promise of humiliation should your little "activity" be discovered is as palpable as ever. Oh, and one more thing: You're no longer in your bathroom. You're in a small "Collection Room" at the doctor's office with your wife, an entire nursing staff, and every single person on the other side of that door knowing *exactly* what you're doing in there.

Suddenly your wife's little "procedures" don't seem nearly as bad anymore, now do they?

Leave Your Ego at the Door

For many men, myself included, the semen analysis test marks a distinct, and potentially deadly, turning point in the fertility process. Till now, it had all been about *her*. *She* needed to have kids. *She* had this problem getting pregnant. *She* required love and support during this most difficult period. Now, for the first time, the doctor will be making direct eye contact with you, and, I can tell you from experience, you'll long for the days when you were being ignored.

When the doctor first mentioned the semen analysis test, I think I refused to take it, or gave my word that I was fine, or some other bullshit like that. To be honest, I even surprised myself with how defensive I became. But the more I thought about it, the more my reaction made sense, and here's why: *If fertility cuts to the very core of what it means to be a woman, then virility cuts to the very core of what it means to be a man.* So to have a virtual stranger not only question that virility but also ask you to *prove* it by masturbating in a cup can be disconcerting, to say the least. Believe me, I get it, I've been there, I know where you're coming from. But here's the God's honest truth: When it comes to infertility treatments, the "real man" isn't the one who can defend his machismo to the bitter end. The real man is the one who can swallow his awkwardness and embarrassment and do what he has to do for the betterment of his family.

I know. Easy in hindsight. But the quicker you come to realize that, the better it will ultimately be for your happiness, your ego and, perhaps most importantly, your marriage.

Getting the Results

DR. ROSEN: In general, the semen analysis test is looking for three things: The sperm quantity, the sperm quality, and the sperm mobility. Low numbers can be temporary (related to stress, illness, some medications, or having sex a few hours before your test) or they can be permanent. Some men either are born without sperm-making capabilities or don't have the right plumbing to connect the testes with the penis. In addition, gonorrhea can sometimes cause the plumbing to scar closed. Some men, but only a small number, go through the male equivalent of menopause and lose the ability to make sufficient sperm for intercourse-related pregnancy. This can be genetically related or due to some kind of toxin from the workplace, home, etc.

The most important thing to do when a semen analysis is abnormal is repeat it. If it is abnormal a second time, it is sound advice to consider seeing a urologist who specializes in male fertility. (Most do not.) A lot of urologists will spend undue time looking for varicoceles, which are nothing more than varicose veins in the scrotum. Whether these cause sperm-related infertility is still debatable, so if your doctor wants to remove a varicocele that he can't feel but can only see with an ultrasound, find another doctor. Also, be prepared for a rectal exam to check your prostrate, seminal vesicles, and vas deferens.

MARC: Yikes! Let's move on.

7

THE ROOM

Remember in chapter 4, when I said that fertility clinics are designed solely for women? Well, that's only because I didn't want to scare you. In fact, there is one room, way in the back (it's always way in the back) that was constructed specifically with the husband in mind. It's the first thing men will ask about when they enter the office and the last thing they'll ever want to see. Of course I'm talking about the dreaded Semen Collection Room. And as further proof that this book is different from every other infertility book out there . . . I'm going to devote a whole damn chapter to it!

So without further ado, here's everything you never wanted to know about that scary little room at the end of the hall with the great big KNOCK BEFORE ENTERING! sign posted outside.

Oh, and one quick caveat before I begin: A lot of what I'll be discussing here is . . . well . . . gross. Just like most everything else in the fertility world. So the sooner you can put aside your inhibitions and say the word "masturbation" without cringing or laughing, the easier all this is going to be for everyone involved.

The Room in Detail

While all collection rooms are different, there are a few elements that most have in common. For one thing, they're small. Really small. Maybe enough room for a chest of drawers, a small couch or recliner, and a TV stand. (See Fig. 2: "Sloppy, Hand-Drawn Diagram".) I've never been to one of those red-light-district "hooker rooms" in Amsterdam, but I imagine it's a more luxurious version of that. Most collection rooms are also pretty clean (thank goodness). I don't know whose job it is to straighten them up after each "visit," but whoever it is, they're not being paid nearly enough.

As soon as you enter, the first thing you'll want to do is lock the door. Most rooms even have signs instructing you to do so, but I'm sure somewhere along the line some poor sap forgot and got caught, literally, with his pants down. Please don't let this be you.

Once the door is locked, you can take a moment to get more familiar with your surroundings. The idea here is to prepare as much as you can beforehand, so when it comes time to "perform," the only thing you'll

Fig. 2: Sloppy, Hand-Drawn Diagram

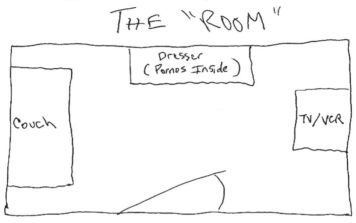

have to think about is your aim. Chances are, the following items will also be available to you:

- **Instruction Sheet.** The nurse may hand it to you beforehand, or you might see a stack of them in plain sight. And no, it doesn't tell you how to jerk off. They figure you know that one already.

- **A Sink.** Wash your hands with the medicinal hospital soap provided. (That's probably number one on the aforementioned instruction sheet.)

- **Paper Towels.** Oh, man, there's an abundance of paper towels (and tissues for that matter).

Chances are you're going to grab a huge handful and wipe down that recliner like you've never wiped anything down before. You'll then spread about a half dozen of them over the recliner, unless of course they provide a disposable paper covering, which many clinics do.

- **Specimen Cups.** You'll see a bunch of them near the sink or on the dresser. You'll want to take one now and label it (clearly!) with all your pertinent information. The instructions will tell you how. I also recommend loosening, or even completely removing, the lid before you begin. You don't want to be fumbling with that at crunch time. Remember, however, that the specimen cup *must* remain sterile, so don't leave it exposed if there's any risk of contamination.

- **Visual Aids.** You'll most likely find a few ratty old porn magazines in a dresser drawer, and a stack of assorted porn DVDs (VHS tapes when I started) on the TV stand. (See next section, "How To Prepare," for more on this.)

- **Collection Slot.** Some of the "better" rooms have a dumbwaiter-like slot where you can leave your sample when you finish. Sometimes it even connects to the embryologists on the other side. This is certainly preferable to the clinics where you have to trudge your specimen cup all the way back to the nurses' station, no doubt passing someone you went to high school with along the way.

How to Prepare

Okay, granted, most guys can walk into that room without reading any of this and do just fine. I mean, it ain't like you haven't been practicing for this moment since you were a kid. But since I have your attention, let me fill you in on some pearls of wisdom that will probably make the whole ordeal a little bit easier and a hell of a lot more productive.

1. Wear "easy" clothes

Trust me. This is not your day to show off those new button-fly jeans or $300 cashmere sweater. You want clothes that are loose fitting, easy to get on and off, and with as few layers as possible. Sweat pants and a T-shirt are the perfect ensemble. I'll even go so far as to say that if you're coming from work, you might want to change into something a bit more comfortable before heading over. There's nothing that can blow an afternoon business deal more quickly than a big glob of jism on your silk Armani power tie.

2. Ask in advance about lubricants

I've heard two schools of thought on this one, and it all comes down to what your specific clinic will allow. Some impose a strict "No Lubricant" policy, while others (the more merciful ones) will permit a small sampling of natural, "nontoxic" lubricants (linseed oil or liquid paraffin, for example) that will not adversely affect a sample. Some will even go so far as to provide you with small vials of the stuff, but if they don't you'll probably want to show up with your own.

3. Consider bringing your own "material"

As I mentioned before, in most of the collection rooms you'll find a small dresser with about a half dozen porno magazines inside. And they're not bad magazines, either. Usually the hard-core variety. Though I guarantee you will be hyper-sensitive to the frayed edges and slight discolorations that are no doubt the handiwork of all the other poor saps who "came" before you. So if you're the kind of guy who feels "icky" when you have to rent used shoes from the bowling alley, then this option is definitely not for you. May I recommend instead the small handful of worn-out DVDs that are scattered around the TV stand in front of you? Again, not a bad selection—but you still might have to contend with a remote control that's been handled a million times by those same poor saps. To be honest, I just always took what was available and lived with it. There was almost something exciting about the element of surprise. But if that's not for you, you're always free to bring your own DVD, press the "play" button with your knuckle, and go.

DR. ROSEN: Not to brag, but in my office all the media is stored on a hard drive (no pun intended), so the only thing people have to touch is the remote, which is contained in a sterile plastic bag. See, guys, I got your back!

4. Store it up good

You know how athletes talk about not having sex before a big game? I never got that. Now, not having sex before a semen analysis test—*that* I get. Remember, the whole purpose of this is to produce a sample that will totally blow away both your wife and your doctor, so a little afternoon delight before heading to the clinic certainly isn't the way to go. Now I'm no expert on this, and I'm too lazy to do the research, but I'd avoid shooting a load for at least 24 hours prior to the test. In fact, go at least two days if you can. That ought to remove anyone's lingering doubt that you're the most John Homes–like virile incarnation of a man to ever step foot in that office.

DR. ROSEN: Given that I am an expert, I can tell you that the real answer is to save up for 36–72 hours.

Other Important Tips

- **Don't miss.** The greatest concentration of sperm is in that first drop, so be sure to aim properly. I can't tell you how many times I screwed this up.

- **Anyone for seconds?** There's no crime in going at it again if you got it in you. It will only make for a larger sample in the long run. (Just be sure to keep the cup sterile if you're using the same one!)

- **Don't joke with nurses.** A lot of guys will want to redirect their nervous energy into humor, but believe me this is neither the time nor the place.

I assure you those nurses out there have heard it all, and you really don't want to be the lucky hundredth guy this month to ask them if they want to "hold your children" when you hand over your sample.

- **Don't be afraid to make suggestions.** Not a good selection of movies? Chair uncomfortable? Say something. Chances are the nurses themselves "designed" these rooms, and I seriously doubt they tested them out beforehand. Not only will they be grateful for the input, but so will you should you ever have to "come" again.

Timing is Everything

It's the age-old question. How long do I stay in there? Too long and they'll wonder what's going on. Too short and they'll think I'm a "quick draw." After more than 30 times in there myself, I can tell you that I've tried it all—stalling, rushing, "double sampling"—and after an exhaustive unofficial study, here's the conclusion I've arrived at: It doesn't make one goddamn lick of difference. Those nurses you're so concerned about are barely even aware of your existence, let alone how long it takes you to rub one out, so just get over yourself.

(With that being said, however, I'd shoot for about 11 minutes, door to door.)

Separating Fact from Fiction

As if jerking off in the cup wasn't bad enough, my test results showed a less-than-stellar sperm count. Nothing that would account for all our infertility problems, but certainly enough to have some impact—maybe 5 to 10 million of the little buggers as compared to the normal 50 million or so. It was at this point that all the usual old wives' tales started to crop up. Wear boxers not briefs, avoid Jacuzzis, stop taking certain medications (in my case, Propecia).

Now, over the past few years I've heard many different experts offer many different opinions as to what does and doesn't work, but as a husband I can tell you this: Do it all. No matter how stupid, no matter how useless. If your wife tells you that her friend's cousin's husband increased his sperm count by jumping up and down in circles, then get yourself a trampoline and start spinning. Whatever it takes (within reason) to keep her happy and keep yourself in her good graces. There's just no reason not to. As I always say—results are good, but avoiding blame is even better.

And for whatever it's worth, my sperm count increased tenfold the next time we checked. So maybe there is something to be said for those uncomfortable boxers after all.

DR. ROSEN: Allow me to address the myths. First off, Propecia. Sorry, Marc, but you lost a million precious hair follicles for nothing. No danger there. However, there are other medications, some high blood pressure pills, for example, that can wreak havoc on the sperm, so it goes without saying you should tell your doctor everything you're on. Heat is another one that's for real. Hot baths, Jacuzzis, saunas, they're all on the fertility blacklist. But when it comes to the underwear myth, all I've got to say is boxers, schmoxers. As long as they aren't skin and air-tight spandex, the type of underwear you wear is completely irrelevant. (Unless of course it's your wife's silk panties, in which case I'm not the type of expert you should be consulting.)

8

GETTING THE RESULTS

Now that you and your wife have been poked, prodded, humiliated, and analyzed, the next big hurdle will be dealing with the results—especially if your doctor discovers a problem. However, as counterintuitive as this may seem, finding something wrong with one or both of you may just be the best news you guys ever get.

Allow me to explain. My wife and I were subjected to all the tests previously mentioned and then some. Even after it all, the experts were really no closer to pinpointing the exact cause of our problem. The official diagnosis was always "unexplained infertility," and, believe me, it is not the diagnosis you want to hear—especially given how many fertility-related ailments are now treatable. (This is particularly true for any male disorders, which, by the way, contribute to roughly 40 percent of infertility cases.)

As an example, I have a friend who—after the aforementioned routine semen analysis—discovered that he was born without a vas deferens (not important what it is) and, as a result, could not ejaculate sperm.

Little more than a decade ago, this would have probably left him and his wife with three choices—sperm donor, adoption, or divorce. However, these days a procedure called intracytoplasmic sperm injection (ICSI) can isolate just one of those precious little sperm and implant it directly into the egg through an in vitro fertilization process. Long story short, he's got two boys now who look just like him.

So to sum it all up, not all diagnoses are surmountable (yet), but knowing what you're up against—and what's required to treat it—is a great step in the right direction.

And if there is a Problem?

Despite my just telling you that "bad news might actually be good news," your wife is still bound to freak out if any abnormalities are discovered. So with that in mind, here are some tips for making both your lives easier when she really starts to lose it.

1. Take an active interest

I can never stress this one enough. During the testing phase, as always, be sure to take an active interest in what's going on. You'd be amazed how much a little "Did that test go well today?" or "Is that a good level?" will calm your wife down and make her feel like she's not in this alone.

2. Focus on the present, not the future

"What if they can't bring my levels down?" "How many years will this set us back?" "Now we'll never get pregnant!" Those are just a few of the many, many things you and your wife will be thinking as the test results start pouring in. Well here's some advice: Don't think those things. As I said in the introduction, the infertility road can be a long one, and a million different factors can affect it, for better or worse, along the way. So the more you avoid projecting every little development on your "ultimate destiny," the saner you'll both be in the long run.

3. Be clear about what is and isn't public information

Everyone's different. Some people benefit from sharing their personal information with others. Some people do not. Now would be a good time for you and your wife to discuss exactly how much of this information gets shared and, perhaps more important, with whom it gets shared.

Take it from me—telling your poker buddies about the "after we screwed" test may seem like a great idea at the time, but I have a sneaking suspicion the wife will think differently.

4. Take the reins with family members

As I explained in chapter 5, your wife's got enough on her plate right now, and the last thing she needs is to worry that your mother is going to ask (again) how "my grandchild" is coming along. So as much as you'd like to play dumb on this one, I'm afraid the time has come to take the reins and nip that sucker in the bud. Don't make a big deal about it. Just casually explain to the relatives in question (hers included) what is and isn't acceptable conversation right now. They may not get it, and if that's the case, then screw 'em. Your loyalty really has to be with your wife right now.

Oh, and one more thing: Use your best judgment as to whether or not you should even tell your wife you took this initiative. As much as you might crave the brownie points, it could (a) just add fuel to the fire, and/or (b) prove much more effective if she thinks these people came to their senses on their own.

5. Get her mind off it

Another one I'll come back to a lot. As this process draws on, you'll discover many times—awaiting test results, charting ovulation, after an IVF procedure—when your wife is playing the "waiting game." This is when your keen ability to distract her should kick into high gear. Find a mutual hobby, suggest a movie, take her on a vacation. Whatever it takes to keep her from "watching the clock."

6. Resist the urge to compare war stories

Yes, we know . . . you had to go into the little room and jerk off to the bad porn while all the giggly nurses waited outside. It's a great story for the afore-mentioned poker buddies (with your wife's permission, of course), but avoid whining to the lady who just had two long tubes and a scope inserted into her abdomen. I'm telling you now, it ain't gonna fly.

7. Avoid the blame game

Remember before your wedding how there was all this talk about "two becoming one," and "now you're a team," and "blessed union of souls" and all that other fun stuff? Well at no time in your marriage will those stupid clichés mean more than during fertility treatments. It's vital that there be no finger-pointing, no fault, no blame. What happens to one of you happens to both of you, and any attitude short of that is disaster. Just ask my buddy with the sperm count so low he could name them all. He was pretty darn happy when his wife didn't blame him, and, believe me, you would be, too.

DR. ROSEN: I'm reminded of a couple I once treated who were obsessed with finding out who was to blame for their infertility (even though the actual causes were unexplained). The question was somewhat answered when the husband, in an attempt to prove his virility once and for all, went ahead and got another woman pregnant! According to the wife (who hysterically relayed the story to me in my office) the husband confessed his sin with a self-satisfied smile and then added, "So I guess it was your fault."

MARC: Now *that's* a bad husband.

Superstitions, Alternative Medicines, and Other Mumbo-jumbo

Right around now, faced with the possibility of expensive procedures and the uncertainty of ever conceiving, is when most women will explore less traditional treatments for infertility, or as your wife will probably call it, some "surefire thing that a friend of a friend swears got her pregnant." This is a pretty far-reaching category, but in general it refers to treatments like acupuncture, holistic medicines, yoga, even prayer. Basically, anything that is not necessarily embraced by the medical community, but is still rumored to have gotten someone, somewhere, pregnant at some time or another. Chances are, your wife has already toyed with at least one of these "cures" by now. It's hard not to with all the information circulating out there, especially on the Internet. In our own case, I can remember as far back as our pre–artificial insemination days having the most God-awful-smelling Chinese root tea brewing on our stove at all hours of the day.

So what's the story with these things? Do they work? To be honest . . . I don't have a frigging clue. However—and this is a big however—if these so-called miracle cures help to calm your wife down and reduce her stress level (which, by the way *has* been proven to make a difference), then by all means let her have her fun. Just so long as it doesn't interfere with, or take the place of, the more proven, scientific methods that we've already discussed. If that happens, then it might be time to have a little talk with her . . . or at least move on to the next section.

ROUND THREE
THE GAME

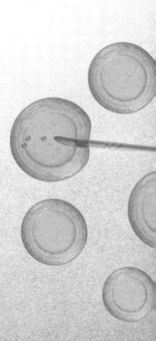

Still not pregnant, huh? That's okay. You've come to the right place. In this section we'll explore the most readily available treatments for infertility sufferers—ranging from the relatively simple *artificial insemination*, to the much more complicated (and stressful, and painful, and expensive) *in vitro fertilization,* to the even more complicated, stressful, and expensive *egg donations, gestational surrogacy, immune therapies.* . . . Okay, I'll just stop there. Any more, and I doubt you'll even turn the page.

9

THE MINOR LEAGUES: STIMULATING DRUGS AND ARTIFICIAL INSEMINATION

Remember in the introduction when I talked about this whole journey being a "process"? Well, leaving the testing phase and entering the treatment phase is certainly one of the bigger steps you guys are going to have to take. In hindsight, I know how relatively simple and painless (both physically and emotionally) many of these initial procedures can be, but that doesn't make the undertaking any less daunting while you're going through them.

Another thing that can be pretty disheartening—and you're really gonna start to sense it about now—is the sheer "artificialness" of it all. As children, we were all taught to believe that conception is an entirely natural process. I don't know about you, but when my parents finally sat me down to discuss the birds and bees, they never said "but if Daddy's sperm or Mommy's eggs are broken, various artificial methods such as intrauterine insemination, ovarian hyperstimulation, or progesterone shots may be necessary." In this chapter we'll explore some of these artificial "baby-making" techniques, and I'll offer up some ways to make the whole thing a bit more bearable and whole lot less awkward.

Fertility Drugs (Wife Psycho Level: 5)

Right about now is when you'll start hearing words that will sound familiar, though you never really knew (or cared about) what they meant. Clomid is probably one of those words, and you're about to learn more about it whether you want to or not.

DR. ROSEN: To quickly break it down, there are generally two types of fertility drugs. One is a pill and the other is a shot. The pill is the aforementioned Clomid, though it can also go by another brand name, Serophene, or its generic name, clomiphene. The shots are called gonadotropins, and there are five different brand names you can buy. (Sorry, no generics, and these puppies are expensive.) They are, in alphabetical order, Bravelle, Follistim, Gonal-F, Menopur, and Repronex.

Clomid

To put it simply (always the best approach), Clomid is a drug that helps your wife ovulate if she has trouble doing so on her own. In some cases it's used to produce more and/or better eggs, but its primary use is for women who don't ovulate at all. The drug is usually taken orally for an average of three to four months and, aside from some possible ultrasounds to monitor the results, requires little other attention.

With that being said, here are some things to keep in mind should your wife start Clomid, or any other ovulation-stimulating drug treatments, for that matter.

- **Multiple Births.** You've probably heard about this one, too. In addition to ripening eggs, these drugs also increase a woman's chances of producing more than one egg each month, which, in turn, increases the likelihood of having more kids. In fact, with Clomid, twins are about 10 percent more likely. And as the father of twins, I can tell you that—while it is a blessing and all that other crap—it is also *more* than twice the work of having just one baby. So please be sure to discuss this important consideration with your wife and your doctor before it happens.

    DR. ROSEN: The downside of multiples isn't only related to the amount of work they require. Having more than one baby in the womb unfortunately increases the risk of birth defects as well.[6] The reason for this is simple. The uterus is designed to feed and nurture only one child at a time, so when more than one is trying to grow in there, two different adverse effects can occur. Some multiples are not able to be nourished properly, which can cause birth defects, and others are born so prematurely that they can acquire problems later on.

- **Hormonal Changes.** Don't you hate that term? It's never good. You never hear that your wife is going through "hormonal changes" that will increase her desire to spend every Sunday planted on the couch with you drinking beer and watching football. It's always these weird, incomprehensible, psycho changes. And yes, those are the very ones she may experience on Clomid. To be more specific, some women (about 20 percent on average) may experience symptoms that are very similar to menopause—hot flashes, headaches, irritability, nausea. Ask your dad about it. Chances are he already went through it with dear old Mom.

---

[6] *The risk of birth defects in a 30-year-old woman are 3 percent for a singleton, 7–8 percent for twins, and 20–30 percent for triplets.*

DR. ROSEN: The reason that Clomid causes these "hormonal changes" is because it works by blocking estrogen. Estrogen is a mood elevator. It makes women feel "good," so if a medication takes away the effect of estrogen, which is what "blocking" means, they don't feel as good. I had one patient who got so depressed and irritable with her husband while she was on Clomid that she went after him with a knife. Good thing he was a Navy SEAL. He told me he had to knock her to the ground to disarm her, but he also told me to never give her that medicine again. Since he was about twice my size, I never did.

- **Anxiety Level.** As with most things related to fertility, your wife will probably freak out when she has to start medication, and there's very little you can do or say to make her feel better about it. In fact, this might be one of the few times when my advice would be to downplay, or even ignore, the treatment rather than draw attention to it. It would be like if you started using Rogaine to grow hair, and every morning your wife asked you if you had any new follicles yet. Considerate, yes, but hardly what you'd want to be reminded of on a daily basis. Your best bet is to just trust she's taking the pills and hope they do their job. Believe me, you'll hear about it eventually either way.

You Got Anything a Little Stronger?

If you and your wife get pregnant on Clomid (as many couples do), consider yourself lucky. Your infertility nightmare has come to a mercifully premature end, and you can now begin the even more nightmarish task of raising children. If, however, Clomid does not work, your doctor will most likely recommend some stronger medication like gonadotropins, which will probably be given as shots.

Again, another hurdle—not so much because of the pain of the needle (hell, that's nothing compared to childbirth), but more because of what it represents to your wife. This isn't mere testing anymore. These are some serious drugs that will be injected into her body. And, rest assured, as the treatments become more aggressive, so do the side effects, and so does the stress level. Just keep that in mind the next time you see your wife crying uncontrollably for "no reason," and cop her a little break if you can.

DR. ROSEN: Here's some good news, though. When it comes to side effects, gonadotropins have far fewer to speak of than Clomid. In fact, some women feel quite good while on them. So what are the potential downsides? Well, the most common is a "bloating feeling" as the eggs ripen. Remember, these medications can ripen 10 to 20 eggs at a time (as opposed to the usual one or two), so the bloating is literally caused by your wife's now bulging ovaries. Other women describe headaches, being tired, or feeling stressed, and some women also complain of increased vaginal discharge that is clear and odorless.

MARC: Hey, watch your language there, Doctor.

DR. ROSEN: Sorry. But if you thought that was scary, check this out: Gonadotropins increase the risk of multiple births to the tune of 20 percent for twins, 5–10 percent for triplets, and a remote possibility of quads or more. And while selective reduction is always an option, the risk of losing all the embryos increases 3–4 percent for each embryo canceled. So, for example, if your wife becomes pregnant with quads, and you elect to abort two of the embryos, there is now a 6–8 percent chance of miscarrying the remaining two embryos as well. Given these factors, it is vital that your doctor closely monitor your wife's egg count (via ultrasound monitoring) during any such treatment, and he may advise stopping cycles (no sex or artificial inseminations) if more than four eggs are present.

Self-Service Injections

I hate needles. I hate seeing them. I hate getting them. I hate so much as thinking about them. So imagine my horror when the doctor suggested that I personally administer these shots to my wife at home. Was he kidding me?! There was about as much chance of that happening as there was me having this baby.

Or so I thought. (The shots part, not the baby part.)

Now, granted, for our first round of injections I held firm and forced my wife to get them at the doctor's office each and every time, but by the time we had progressed to in vitro fertilizations, and the injections were much more frequent, I had no choice but to abandon my fears and give her the shots myself. (I talk about this more in chapter 10, "In Vitro Fertilization.")

So here's the point: If a wimp like me can eventually come around, then you can, too. Feel it out with your wife. Feel it out with your doctor. Weigh all the external factors—do you live far from the doctor's office, can you afford all those appointments, can your wife easily take off from work—and, in the end, if it makes more sense for you to administer the shots, then try to rise to the occasion.

Artificial Insemination (Wife Psycho Level: 2)

In the beginning of this chapter I touched on the "artificial" nature of all these treatments, and the aptly named artificial insemination is certainly no exception. Usually performed in conjunction with the aforementioned stimulation drugs, artificial insemination is a more controlled way of getting your "boys" closer to where they need to go. Think of it as the conception equivalent of "asking for directions," but with even more resistance and discomfort on your part.

DR. ROSEN: I'd like to get a little more technical here if I could. Normally, when a couple has sex, about 50–100 million motile sperm get into the vagina, and within seconds, a few million of them are pulled up into the uterus. From there, the sperm are pumped up to and then through the fallopian tubes to get to the egg. By contrast, an intrauterine (artificial) insemination is a process where sperm are placed directly into the uterus. There is one problem with this, though. You can't put semen directly into the uterus, because the semen contains hormones called prostaglandins that would literally cause the uterus to turn itself inside out. The solution, therefore, is to remove these hormones prior to the insemination in a process called "sperm washing" (another term you might have heard before). Once the sperm have been washed—once the wheat has been separated from the chaff—they can be inserted into the uterus with a small, soft plastic tube. This is usually easy and virtually pain free.

As you might have already guessed, the first step to performing this relatively simple procedure is acquiring the little guys in the first place, and, yes, that will require another trip to the dreaded "Room." However, if you live close enough to the doctor, you might also ask about producing a sample at home and delivering it right to the office. More than likely, the doctor will be okay with this, just so long as it's collected in exactly the same manner (sterile cup, no lubricant, no spillage) and is delivered to the office NO MORE than 45 minutes later.

I gotta be honest. I always preferred the "delivery" method, if for no other reason than I would intentionally speed like a motherf**ker to the doctor's office just begging for a cop to stop me. I couldn't imagine a more perfect excuse than "Please officer [hold up cup], this is a sample of my semen that has to be delivered to a doctor in less than a half hour, or a month's worth of preparation to finally conceive will be ruined. [Hold up cup again. Stare at it wistfully.] My children's lives depend on this." Sadly, I never got pulled over (it figures), but if I was, I doubt there's a cop out there who would ticket me. Please try it yourself, and let me know if it works.

Staying the Course vs. Moving On

Over a two-year period, my wife and I subjected ourselves to 16 artificial inseminations and an equal number of painful, and potentially dangerous, rounds of stimulation drugs. Why so many? Well, for starters, we got pregnant on the first go-round (though we eventually miscarried) and were determined to recapture that early success. For another, we were justifiably petrified of moving up to the next level of treatment—in vitro fertilizations—and were hoping against hope that the next artificial insemination would be the winner.

Both of these were lousy reasons. And I can't stress enough how important it is to trust your gut (and your doctor) enough to know when any phase of the process has run its course. Because after a while, you will just be "spinning your wheels."

DR. ROSEN: As we mentioned before with natural conception as well as with Clomid, three to four treatment cycles is plenty. The hard part comes when you con-

ceive and then miscarry on cycle number 4. Do you do four more before moving on? The answer is maybe. Most doctors would ask you to do at least two to three more before you go on to the next step.

But what if my wife and I disagree?

This is, in many ways, a rhetorical question, because the fact is you *will* disagree. It's inevitable. You're two distinct individuals—each with your own opinions, your own timetables, and your own thresholds for this particular kind of pain—so I can all but guarantee that the day will come (many days in fact) when one of you will want to give it another go (most likely her) and the other will want to throw in the towel (most likely you). The trick, of course, is to work through those disagreements with as little collateral damage as possible and, to that end, here are a few hard-learned pearls of wisdom that helped keep my sanity and my marriage intact.

1. Pick your battles

Like anything else in life, there are the issues that matter and the issues that MATTER. Just be sure to stick to the great big capital-lettered ones and let those measly little lowercase ones fall by the wayside. Giving your wife injections, jerking off in cups, charting your sex life—these are inconveniences, to be sure, but hardly the stuff of deal breakers. (Easy for me to say now, right?) Remember, every time you make a stink or refuse to do something unpleasant, it puts another chink in the armor of your marriage, so just be sure not to strip too much of it away before the heavy artillery even rolls out.

I remember one particularly heinous test they wanted to give me that required swabbing the inside (that's right, inside) of my penis with a thin metal Q-tip-like thingy.[7] (Did you squirm just now? Betcha did.) Needless to say, I freaked. Actually I more than freaked. I put my foot down and said I would rather never have kids than subject myself to that. I held out for weeks, drove my wife crazy, and then finally, with the aid of

---

[7]In case you're wondering, they were testing for, of all things, a venereal disease called chlamydia. It was a required part of the workup I had to do before they would implant our embryos in a surrogate. I desperately tried to convince my wife, our lawyers, and the surrogate's family that there was no way I had chlamydia, but somehow my word just wasn't gonna cut it this time.

about three drinks and a half a Valium, dropped trou for the admittedly unpleasant couple of seconds. So what did I gain by this little hissy fit? Absolutely nothing. In fact, all I did was lower my street cred when it came to the differences of opinion that really mattered.

2. Avoid sweeping assertions

When confronted with life-altering decisions like in vitro fertilization, surrogacy, or adoption, it's only natural to get somewhat adamant and defensive about your opinions. I WILL do this, I would NEVER do that, over my dead body would that EVER happen. Yet as much as you believe those things in the moment, it's important to remember that the infertility process is long, and it's complicated, and it's ever changing. So, as much as possible, try to avoid making sweeping assertions that may very well shift over time. If you had asked me early on in our journey if I would do half the crap we did, I would have said, "No friggin' way!" But attitudes change, lines in the sand are moved, and adjustments are made. Desperation has a way of doing that to you. So

before you go shouting "Never!" consider soften-
ing that to an "I'm not there yet." Because, more
often than not, it's not so much your beliefs that
are different—just your degrees of readiness.

3. See the forest for the trees

Okay, first off, how dumb an expression is that?
It doesn't make sense grammatically or even
metaphorically, but its meaning—to see the bigger picture—does apply well here. Often, in the
throes of infertility hell, we get so caught up in
the moment that we don't stop and think about
how our split-second-impulse decisions can have
long-term effects on both our lives and our marriage. So before you go putting the kibosh on any
more testing, or adamantly refuse to pay for an
in vitro fertilization, consider the toll—in anger,
in resentment, in bitterness—those choices can
take, not only today but well into the future. For
myself there was always a simple litmus test. If
my wife wanted something more than I *didn't*
want it, then I would graciously step aside and let
her have her way. People often saw that as loving
and selfless. I merely saw it as self-preservation.

4. There's a time and a place for everything

We all have strong opinions and eventual break-ing points. That's fine. But at least be somewhat smart about where and when you let them be known, especially given how fragile and sensi-tive your wife is right now. If you have an ax to grind or a beef to pick (two more baffling idi-oms), find a time when the two of you are alone with little distraction and no additional stress. Don't make a stand in a restaurant, or at a party (God forbid a baby shower), or when she just got home from a long day at work. Show her that you at least thought this out enough to "do it right." I have my own cautionary tale about this one. Maybe my biggest faux pas of all. It was when our surrogate was being implanted with our embryos. We were all in the doctor's office —me, my wife, the surrogate—and just as the doctor was about to insert those four seeds of life into the surrogate's body, I turned to my nervous wife and whispered "This better work, 'cause you're done."

I'll never live that one down. Never.

5. Find an objective voice

Here's the thing: There's no right and wrong in all this. If your wife gets pregnant, she was a genius to undergo so many risky procedures. If she doesn't, she was a fool to try. Obviously that makes any argument to the contrary both tricky and completely subjective, so it may help to find an objective voice to step in and moderate. And by "objective voice," I don't mean your buddy at work or your wife's mother. Everybody has his or her cheering section who are there to tell them they're right, and that's all well and good. But by all means don't use these people as ammunition to defend your point, or take their word as the gospel truth. Save that for a professional, be it one-on-one counseling or a support group led by someone trained in these areas. You may not find all the answers or solve all your issues, but at least you'll be one step closer to finding a common ground.

I'd like to say I followed all my advice, and my wife and I never had so much as a squabble. Sadly, that wasn't the case for us or, I imagine, for anyone going through this. The most any of us can hope for is to grow from the experience and, with any luck, come out the other side stronger and more in touch with each other than when we began. I've heard it said that infertility can either make your marriage stronger or tear it apart, and for the most part I believe that to be true. There's no guaranteeing which category you'll fall into, but your eventual success or failure does have an awful lot to do with the choices you make along the way.

Speaking of choices, my wife and I had an important one to make right about now. We had exhausted fertility drugs, exhausted artificial inseminations, and we were plain old exhausted. Still with nothing to show for our efforts and my wife's 35th birthday rapidly approaching, we bit the bullet and moved one more rung up the ladder—to the dreaded in vitro fertilization. As always, we figured it would just be one time. As always, we were grossly mistaken. Thankfully, for the sake of our sanity, we didn't know that at the time.

10

THE MAJOR LEAGUES:
IN VITRO FERTILIZATION

I won't lie to you. In vitro fertilization (IVF for short) is a bitch. Physically, psychologically, financially— there ain't nothing fun about this sucker (which, by the way, rates a solid 8 on the Wife Psycho Level.) And you want some more good news? It might not even work. In fact, a woman's chances of conceiving a baby through IVF (with her own eggs) at age 35 are about 35–50 percent. At 42 her chances drop to 10 percent. After 45 they're pretty much nil.[8] To put it in perspective, imagine going to Vegas and dropping $10,000 at the Big Six Wheel (which, at 40%, offers the worst odds of any casino game). People would think you were nuts! And

---

[8]For the record, the chances of conceiving naturally during a given menstrual cycle should never exceed 25 percent (even for a woman in her twenties), and will drop well below 10 percent after the age of 40. So as dire as the in vitro numbers appear, they still up the odds considerably.

yet, that's pretty much what you're doing every time you roll the dice on an IVF treatment.

So why do it? Because at this stage of the game, it's still the best chance you've got for having your own biological child. It's not a miracle cure, for sure. But then again, it's a hell of a lot more opportunity than your parents' generation had.

In this chapter we'll explore the many facets of in vitro fertilization. What it is, how it works, and how it can ultimately affect you, your wife, and your relationship. This is the big league, folks. And if there was ever a procedure that could ultimately test the strength of your character and your relationship, you're about to walk smack dab into it.

DR. ROSEN: In fact, the chances of getting pregnant through IVF are related to a number of separate issues. These include the skill of your doctor, the skill of his laboratory, the age of your wife, the quality of her eggs, and how many times you've tried IVF before. Thankfully, however, the quality of your sperm matters very little. As long as you've got some, you're pretty much a go.

What is "In Vitro Fertilization"?

Like Clomid, I'm guessing IVF is another term you've vaguely heard of but never knew anything about. You probably also remember hearing about Louise Brown, the world's first "Test Tube Baby," when you were a kid and tuning out (as I did) once you realized that she didn't *really* grow up inside a test tube. In fact, Brown, now in her thirties and a mother herself, was the first successful in vitro fertilization birth and ushered in the million plus IVF babies who came after her.

So why the term "Test Tube Baby"? Well, for one thing, it looks really good in a headline. But beyond that, it (loosely) refers to the fact that, unlike natural conception, or even artificial insemination for that matter, IVF babies are conceived entirely outside the womb. That's right. A *truly* immaculate conception where even a virgin can carry her own biological child to term. Now that's what I call holding out.

"So How Does it All Work? (In 200 Words or Less, Please.)"

You ever try to fix an appliance without taking it apart first? You kind of fish your hands around inside and feel for the faulty wire or the loose screw and hope you get it right? Well, that's sort of what's happening when the doctor tries to "fix" your fertility issues with stimulation drugs or artificial inseminations. Sure, he (or she) might tap into the problem immediately and fix it right then and there, but in a sense, he's still flying blind.

Now imagine instead if he could take the parts outside the machine and work directly on them in a more controlled environment. Well, that's exactly what's going on in an IVF treatment. Anywhere from 1 to 30 eggs (depending on how many can be produced in a single cycle) are surgically extracted from your wife, and the best ones are then fertilized in a petri dish with your recently collected sperm (yeah, it's back to The Room again). The resulting embryos are then closely observed in the lab for anywhere between three and five days, at which point the best of these are reimplanted into your wife to (with any luck) grow into a baby. See, it's *simple*! (And for those of you not counting, that was exactly 200 words.)

Your Wife the Drug Addict

You may have wondered why I spoke so casually about your wife's drug intake up until this point. Easy. I went through 10 IVF treatments. And compared to that shit, everything else before it looks like Flintstone multivitamins. Seriously, guys, you will not believe the amount of medication that's required to complete an IVF cycle.

Here's a word: Lupron. Remember it. You'll be hearing it a lot. Lupron is a drug that shuts down the messages from your wife's brain that tell her to produce one egg every month. When it is combined with other drugs that stimulate egg production, as many as 30 can be produced in a single cycle. I think our personal record was 27.

DR. ROSEN: There's a common misconception that a woman will enter early menopause if so many eggs are retrieved at once, and it's simply not true. In fact, a healthy woman in her twenties and early thirties has 40–50 eggs available each month, though nature normally allows for only one to ovulate while the other 39–49 die from lack of food. In order to "produce" this many eggs at one time, we are merely nourishing more of that existing monthly supply that would otherwise not survive anyway.

In addition to turning your wife into a human bunny, Lupron also helps keep her from ovulating too early—a very important thing given how controlled an IVF cycle has to be. Your doctor may also prescribe additional drugs like Antagon or Cetrotide (in lieu of Lupron), which are specifically designed to suppress ovulation.

Throughout it all, your wife will be monitored by her doctor on a near-daily basis. More often than not, this will require a steady stream of blood tests and ultrasounds to determine if the drugs are doing their job properly or if any adjustments need to be made. As I mentioned earlier, this is as good a reason as any to choose a doctor close to your home. Your wife will be under enough stress right now. She doesn't need to add freeway rush-hour traffic to the mix.

After about ten days of this madness, your wife will be asked to take her hCG shot. Never heard of it? Oh, you will, my friend. You will. HCG stands for human chorionic gonadotropin (don't worry, you won't be tested on this stuff), and its job is simple. This is the drug that finally tells your wife's body to release all those eggs so they can be retrieved for fertilization. It's like the green flag in racing, the starting gun in track, the snap in football. And it's administered about 35 hours before the retrieval is scheduled to take place.[9]

DR. ROSEN: Patients often ask about the timing of the hCG shot—why it's always 35 hours before the egg retrieval—and the reason has to do with maturation vs. ovulation. Take the eggs too early, and they will not be mature enough to fertilize. Take them too late, and they will have already begun to ovulate, in which case we

---

[9]The hormone that a woman's body normally produces to cause ovulation is called "luteinizing hormone," or LH. The body is unable to differentiate between LH and hCG, and hCG is currently a lot cheaper to administer.

won't be able to find them anymore. The analogy I often use is picking fruit. Pick too early, and the fruit never ripens. Too late, and it's already rotten. So, in the case of egg retrieval, at least, that magic number for perfect "picking" translates to 35 hours after the eggs have been exposed to hCG.

A word of warning about the hCG shot: Because of this crucial timing, your wife will be insane with taking the shot *exactly* 35 hours before her scheduled egg retrieval. (And it doesn't help that 35 hours before the retrieval usually translates to the middle of the night.) She will mention it incessantly, she will set about three alarm clocks, she will make sure all the flashlights in the house are working in case there's a blackout. Just go with it, guys. Smile, nod, think about baseball. The lady's nervous and stressed out. You can't blame her, really.

So all These Drugs are Administered Orally, Right?

Yes, of course. They're a little bitter, though, so be sure to tell your wife to mix them with Kool-Aid or Tang if she—

What, are you nuts! They're shots, man! Long, awful, painful shots like you used to get as a kid. The kind that made you scream until you passed out when you finally realized why your mom and the doctor were being so nice to you all of a sudden. And get this? You are going to be expected to give these shots.

I know. That's insane. I thought so, too, when the nurse first brought it up. I felt like Karen Black in *Airport '75* when she was asked to land that crippled 747. And I wouldn't even have George Kennedy in the tower to talk me down!

Here's the thing, though. Agreeing to stick your wife with a relentless series of powerful and painful injections is perhaps the most thoughtful and romantic gesture you can offer her right now. No, really. This is your opportunity to step up to the plate and say "I know what you're going through, and I want to help. I want to be a part of it." As opposed to what I said, which was more along the lines of "No friggin' way. I'd rather adopt."

So how did I finally come around? Not easily, I can assure you. At first, I insisted my wife get her shots at the doctor's office every day. And I mean *every day*. Sometimes more than once a day. I also sat idly by when, in a fit of desperation, she attempted to do it herself—fairly successfully for the smaller shots in her belly, but much less successfully for the big ones in her butt. I let her call friends, and even hired a professional nurse when no one else could be found.

Then, finally, thankfully, I agreed to let the nurse teach me what to do. I learned how to load the plunger with the medication. I listened to where and how the injection should be administered. I practiced on an orange, which apparently has the same consistency as human skin and muscle. And finally I watched as the nurse drew a Magic Marker bull's-eye on my wife's ass to show me exactly where to aim. (No joke. It's done a lot.)

I'd love to tell you that after a while I became more comfortable with it, but I can't. If anything, it only became more unpleasant as her skin started to harden and scar from all the days of abuse. I'd also love to tell you I got consistently better at it, but I can't tell you that either. In fact, on the very last shot I gave, I hit my wife's sciatic nerve and left her limping for about three weeks. Maybe that's because I never looked. Never, not once. I would pick a spot, make a mental image, close my eyes, and go.

I did it. Poorly, I grant you, but I did it all the same. And while I in no way want to compare the pain I went through to the pain my wife went through, we were still sharing in the pain. As warped and messed up as that might sound, it did help to bring us closer together.

DR. ROSEN: With all due respect to Marc, the aforementioned "long, awful, painful shots" aren't nearly as long, awful, or painful as they used to be. In fact, most of the injections prior to the egg retrieval can now be given with a very thin half-inch needle in the abdomen. There is, however, one shot that is still given with a one-and-a-half-inch needle in the hip or upper buttock. This has not changed.

MARC: And that shot would be?

DR. ROSEN: Progesterone, a shot that's started after the egg retrieval.

MARC: See! So it's still no walk in the park, guys.

Are there any possible side effects?

Now, really . . . what do you think the chances are that there wouldn't be side effects? Of course there are side effects! Some physical. Some emotional. All terrible. On the physical side we have bloating, headaches, and skin breakouts, just to name a few. On the emotional side we have mood swings, hot flashes, and all the aggravation she's going to feel from those aforementioned physical side effects. And that doesn't even begin to address the stress level, financial burden, and sheer panic of doing an IVF treatment in the first place.

Now, I got lucky. While my wife experienced many of the aforementioned side effects and then some, she never had the kind of severe mood swings that other husbands have reported back to me. I'm talking some serious "crazy girl" mood swings, the likes of which you've never seen before. Even worse than that seemingly fun-loving girl in college who started to bawl uncontrollably when you tried to have sex with hcr for the first (and last) time. It's not like your wife is going to admit to these side effects, either. No, I'm afraid when she lashes out at you and calls you a prick for absolutely nothing, she will adamantly, 100 percent, stand by her feeling that you're a prick. And if you dare try to explain that it's the medication talking, she'll call you a fucking prick.

In case you haven't figured it out yet . . . this is a bad two weeks.

So What Can I do About It?

Finally, a good question. I only wish I had a good answer. The truth is, there isn't much you can do except ride it out the best you can. If you sense your wife needs comfort, comfort her. If you sense she wants to talk about it, bring it up. If you sense she wants her space, by all means leave her alone. This is one of the few times when you might have a better idea of what your wife wants and needs than even she does, so use your best judgment.

I say again . . . no marriage is left untouched by infertility. Either it is made stronger or it is made weaker. And rest assured, the power is within you to decide which way it goes.

The Retrieval

What could be better than nearly two weeks of painful injections and sheer misery? Oh, I don't know . . . how about surgery? Sure, that sounds good!

About twelve days after this hell begins, and exactly 35 hours after the aforementioned hCG shot, you'll find yourself wheeling your wife on a stretcher down a surgical-center or hospital corridor, telling her everything will be all right and hoping to God that it really will.

And what will you be doing while your wife is being put under general anesthesia and having two years' worth of eggs surgically extracted from her body all at once? You guessed it, dude. It's back to The Room for perhaps the worst, most unsatisfying orgasm you will ever have in your entire life. And that includes the crazy college chick I mentioned a few paragraphs back.

Making an Embryo

So she did the drugs, they took her eggs, you gave your sperm. Now the only thing left to do is make an embryo, and that's where the aptly named embryologist comes in. If you never met one of these remarkable men (or women) before, let me describe him to you. By and large, he was that nerdy kid in biology class who sat in the first row and reminded the teacher when it was time for a quiz. You might have even pummeled the ass of someone just like him back in grade school. Let's just hope it wasn't on the day he was supposed to learn how babies were made.

In order to fully appreciate how important the embryologist is to an IVF treatment, imagine him as the general manager of a professional football team. (Something, I guarantee you, he has never been.) Like any good GM, it's his job to create the best team possible from all the available players. In this case, he'll start with the defense—also known as eggs. Out of the 20 or so recruits, a few will be cut immediately. Too mature, not mature enough, lacking a chromosome or two, you know the drill. After carefully observing the rest of the lineup over a 24-hour period, the best of the best will be drafted for play, and the rest will be left crushed and destroyed (literally).

Now it's time to call up all those offensive sperm cells who have been waiting patiently on the bench. In a sort of "open tryout," the whole lot of them will take to the field, also known as a petri dish, and enter into a fierce skirmish with the defensive eggs. Most will be eliminated early on, but a few lucky players will rise to the occasion and prove an equal match to their defensive counterparts. There is one exception to this, however. If the number of sperm cells proves inadequate (remember my friend without the vas deferens), then open tryouts are canceled and one single sperm will be chosen as an early draft pick. (See ICSI back in chapter 8).[10]

Over the next three to five days, your fertility doctor and embryologist will keep a close eye on all these growing embryos and report back to you and your wife at regular intervals. Ideally you're looking to have as many eight-cell embryos as possible on the third day, at which point they can be safely reimplanted back into your wife.[11]

---

[10]For those of you too lazy to flip back a few pages, ICSI is when one individual sperm is isolated and then injected directly into the egg (with a glass needle that is only about 50 percent bigger in diameter than the head of the sperm).

[11]On average, 50 percent of three-day-old embryos will be of good quality for a 30-year-old woman, as opposed to only 20 percent for a 38-year-old woman.

Quality Vs. Quantity

As you've probably guessed, the quality of these embryos holds far greater importance than their quantity. (Likewise for the individual eggs and sperm before them.) Using my own experiences as an example, I can remember some IVF treatments that yielded 20-plus embryos with only 5 usable ones, and other IVF treatments with less than 10 embryos, but all were worthy candidates. Just a friendly reminder for when your wife starts bitching because her friend produced more embryos than she did.

Alternatively, if the embryos are really thriving, the doctor may suggest waiting till the fifth day and perform what's called a *blastocyst transfer.* The advantage to a blastocyst transfer is that the resulting embryos have a much greater chance of survival after the transfer. The disadvantage is that some or all may not survive to the fifth day, and then you're screwed. Assuming your doctor is a good one, he or she will spell out all the pros and cons so you can make the most educated decision possible. Again, this is why having a good rapport with the fertility doctor is so vitally important.

DR. ROSEN: Another advantage of blastocyst transfer is that fewer embryos can be transferred without decreasing your chances of having a child. Transferring fewer embryos means fewer triplets and quadruplets.

MARC: Always a good thing!

Yes, You Can Love One Kid More.

With any luck you've now got 10 to 15 embryos with varying degrees of quality. Using a very specific grading scale, your doctor and/or embryologist will tell you the viability of each and every one of them and even show you pictures for good measure. Think of it as your very first parent-teacher conference!

Now it's time to decide how many of the little guys to put back in Mom, and chances are your immediate response will be "All of them." I mean, hell, you paid for them, right? Why shouldn't you get your money's worth? However, before you go treating an embryo transfer like the early-bird special at Hometown Buffet, you might want to consider one thing: As unlikely as it is to happen, every one of those embryos has the potential to become a baby. And unless you're willing to "selectively reduce" (you know, abort) some of those embryos after the fact, then you very well might end up like those poor schmucks on the news with the six tiny babies who inevitably have one or two rejects among them, or, worse yet, like Octomom. Also keep in mind that you can probably freeze any remaining embryos "for later," although this can get costly—to the tune of a few hundred, or even thousand, bucks per year, depending on how many batches you have. (For the record, I think we still have six kids frozen on ice in two different states. It was more, but I stopped paying for the kids in New Jersey. Talk about your deadbeat dads.)[12]

Obviously deciding how many embryos to transfer is a very personal decision with no right or wrong answer. Moral, ethical, and religious beliefs will certainly come into play, as will more obvious factors such as your wife's age, her fertility history, and your mutual ability and/or desire to go through this nightmare again if it doesn't work. In the end, these are choices that you are going to have to make as a couple, but more often than not, your doctor will also help steer you toward the most appropriate decision.

My wife and I usually transferred the best four and froze the rest. Given the rising success rates for IVF in the past few years, however, that number would probably be high today. The Society for Assisted

---

[12]So what happens to frozen embryos you no longer want? In general, you have three choices. Destroy them, donate them to research, or give them away to another couple in need. My hope was to harvest their stem cells for new hair, but apparently that's not legal or something.

Reproductive Technology currently recommends that only one or two embryos be transferred on your first attempt at IVF if you are under 40, and three to four only if you're over 40, as the risk of twins and triplets is far less at this age.

Moving Back In with Mom

Okay, here's the good news. Putting those fertilized embryos back inside your wife will be a hell of a lot easier than it was to take her eggs out. In fact, an embryo transfer really isn't that different from your old artificial insemination days (assuming you don't count all the additional time, money, and stress). As during that procedure, your wife will lie down on the table and spread her legs in that medieval-looking device. The doctor will then insert the embryos through her cervix and into the uterus via a catheter and—voilà!—that will be $10,000 please.

Okay, so maybe it's a little more complicated than that. And certainly more stressful. Truth be told, the more you can downplay this day and all it represents, the better off you'll be. Stress does play a part in this, guys. It plays a huge part. More than your wife will ever admit to. Why do you think so many couples get pregnant right after they adopt? Because the pressure's off, the stress level goes down, and suddenly she's able to conceive. And nowhere is this more readily apparent than when your wife tenses up during an embryo transfer.[13]

"It All Went Great!"

These four simple words were the kiss of death in nearly all our embryo transfers. You see, as a couple with unexplained infertility, there was no reason for everything not to go great. We had great eggs. We had great sperm. We had great embryos. We had great transfers. We had no baby! So if you hear those words, please just take them with a grain of salt. Sure, it beats having the doctor throw his speculum to the ground and shout, "Why the hell did I order that third martini at lunch?" But by the same token, this is a very inexact science, and you'd be well served to not put all your hopes on a few encouraging words.

---

[13]A 2004 study conducted by the University of San Diego found that women who were unduly stressed about the medical aspects of IVF had 20 percent fewer eggs retrieved and 19 percent fewer eggs fertilized than women who were less inclined to stress about it.

I know telling your wife to "stop stressing" is much easier said than done. But whatever you can do to calm her, distract her, make her laugh, the greater your chances that this whole thing will go off without a hitch. As best you can, try to think of yourselves as airline passengers with a very skilled and well-trained pilot at the helm. You wouldn't stress out about what controls he was using, or if he put the flaps down, or if he studied the flight plan. He's a professional, for God's sake. He knows what he's doing. Well, guess what? So does the doctor. So as much as is humanly possible, the two of you should just sit back, let the man do his job, and focus instead on where the hell that $10,000 is going to come from.

The 12 Days from Hell (Wife Psycho Level: 9)

With the embryo transfer now behind you, I'd love nothing more than to say the hardest part is over. But I can't. In fact the hardest part lies just ahead of you, my friend. And the reason for that can be boiled down to just one word. Waiting. You see, just because the embryos went in, doesn't mean they're gonna stay in. And unfortunately it will be another long and stressful twelve or so days before an official pregnancy can be confirmed.

Looking back on everything my wife and I went through (and, as you know, we went through a lot), I think this period of time was probably the most traumatic, if for no other reason than that we felt so helpless. She, because there was no more active role for her to take (as I said before, she was the Doer's Doer), and me because I didn't have a clue how to make her feel better.

In the end, there isn't much you *can* do to make her feel better. It is what it is. However, with that being said, here are a few simple tips that might help take the edge off.

1. Let her vent

"I'm pregnant." "I'm not pregnant." "I feel a twinge." "I feel nothing." "My breasts are sore, so it worked!" "I'm spotting, so it didn't work!" These are just a few of the many things your wife will say as she obsesses, questions, second-guesses, mulls, ruminates, doubts, and rejoices all at the same time. And when I say all at the same time, I mean all at the same time. I remember my wife once crying hysterically because she was 100 percent sure that the transfer didn't work, and she hadn't even designed the nursery yet! They're crazy. At this point even they'll admit they're crazy. So instead of arguing about it or trying to put a stop to it, your best plan of attack is to just let her vent. After all, it isn't like she's really talking to you anyway. I know it *sounds* like she's talking to you—what with her looking right at you and speaking and all. But the truth is, she's just using you as a sounding board for all these millions of thoughts that she has to say out loud or she'll implode. So—as always—just nod, smile politely, and say whatever the hell it is that she wants to hear. It will all be over soon, I promise.

2. Get her mind off it

Let me rephrase that. Do whatever you can, in whatever small way, to get her mind off it for even a second. Talk about current events, a funny thing that happened at work—really anything that doesn't involve babies, pregnancy, or parenthood. At this point, you might wonder if such topics even exist in your world anymore, but wrack your brains and I'm sure you'll come up with something.

3. Keep her away from things that upset her

As I mentioned in chapter 2, there are certain obvious triggers—babies and pregnant women, children's clothing stores, other people's kids—that are like an infertile woman's kryptonite. Plain and simple—keep her away from this shit at all costs. During one particularly harrowing 12-day period, I thought it would be a really great idea to take my wife to Disneyland to get her mind off the whole thing. Suffice to say, the Mad Hatter didn't hold a candle to my wife's level of crazy on that day.

4. Steer her toward things that please her

While my Disneyland idea was grossly ill conceived, I was at least on the right track. More than likely your wife will want to spend the entire 12 days hermited up in the house like some sort of childless Howard Hughes (which would be a much better analogy if Howard Hughes hadn't died childless). Regardless, this would definitely be a good time to remind your wife of all the things she loves to do—be it hobbies, going to the movies, pampering herself, or travel, just to name a few. Maybe even plan a trip in advance just so she has something to look forward to. This might also be a good time to remind her how much she loved those fertility support groups.

5. Pregnancy tests

Inevitably your wife will want to take a home pregnancy test (or seven) before it's time to check her blood at the doctor's office. Most experts will advise not to do this because it's probably too early to show a positive result, but I say that's all the more reason to go for it. This way if, by some miracle, it comes up positive—great. If, however, it comes up negative, you can always blame it on the timing—"See, I told you it was too soon!"—and no one is the worse for wear.

But At Least The Shots are Over, Right?

Oh jeez, I guess you didn't get the memo on this one. While it's true that you won't have to give those awful Lupron shots anymore, I'm afraid they've been replaced by the more awful progesterone shots to help maintain the pregnancy. And why are they more awful? Mostly because their oil-based consistency makes them that much more difficult to give and that much more painful to receive. As I said before, guys . . . the hardest part is far from over.

DR. ROSEN: While progesterone shots are still widely used, there are, for better or worse (depending on your tastes), some alternatives. Many programs have switched to a vaginal pill called Endometrin, which contains micronized progesterone that dissolves like Pop Rocks in the woman's vagina. Alternately there is a rather unpleasant medication called Crinone (Cry None, get it?) that's like putting toothpaste in the vaginal canal with a straw and plunger to get the pasty stuff inside. Some women love the pills or paste, while others would just as soon stick to shots to avoid all the intravaginal leakage and mess.

MARC: Wow. That was particularly gross. Even for you.

Getting the Results

Did I mention we did nine of these things? That's right, nine IVF treatments—but even more important, nine failed IVF attempts.[14] I cannot begin to describe to you the feeling of futility when you reach the end of this road and have nothing to show for it. Truly, nothing. In

---

[14]Technically we did 10 IVFs, but the last one was in conjunction with our surrogate. More on that in chapter 12.

fact, if anything, you just have another black mark on your record for the next time.

If there'll even be a next time.

Now, this isn't to say that the procedure will necessarily fail. If that were the case, nobody would even attempt it in the first place. It's just that . . . well . . . as I said before, your odds at the Big Six Wheel in Vegas are still better than your odds of having a successful in vitro fertilization. So if you're one of the lucky 30 percent or so, congratulations! It was hard, but you did it. If, however, you're among the less fortunate two-thirds of us, please read on.

11

A SWING AND A MISS: WHAT TO DO IF IT DOESN'T WORK

This won't be a very long chapter. There really isn't all that much I can say. Except this: Few things will ever be as devastating, for either of you, as failing that first IVF treatment. And while no single piece of advice can make things all better, I can at least offer a few tips to avoid making things worse. (All of which, by the way, I learned the hard way.)

Don't Downplay Failure. It is a Big Deal.

Your instinct at this point might be to put on a good face and "shrug it off" for her, but I strongly discourage you from doing that. Now more than ever, your wife needs someone she can share her grief with. She needs to know that you, like her, are experiencing a sense of loss and a sense of fear. Maybe not to the same extent, and maybe not for the same reasons, but as her partner you must empathize all the same.

In my own case, the fear and the loss weren't so much a result of the failed IVF as of seeing how much she was suffering because of it. Sure I was upset. Who wouldn't be? But just as I wanted kids, and she *needed* kids, I wanted this IVF to work . . . and she *needed* it to work. In your own case, now that it hasn't worked, at least acknowledge the devastation that setback will undoubtedly cause.

This isn't to say you should be pessimistic or, dare I even say it, fatalistic. That attitude can still be reserved exclusively for her. I just don't want you to downplay the magnitude of this setback. That will only make her feel worse.

Flowers Might Not be the Answer

Around our sixth unsuccessful IVF, my wife was good enough to tell me to stop marking the occasion with flowers. They didn't make her feel better. They were just another reminder of how she had failed—sent more out of pity then anything else. I suspect it wasn't much different from how I felt when she would "sweet-talk" me into procreation sex. Flattered, appreciative, but no less aware of what's really going on here.

Now, every woman is different. Your wife might love flowers (or some other kind of gift). It might be just what she needs to get her out of her funk. I can only speak for myself. And I can tell you that, at least after a while, the well-intentioned gesture did more harm than good.[15]

No One is to Blame

There's an episode of *The Simpsons* in which Homer, in desperate need of cash, suggests that Marge become a surrogate mother. When she refuses, he shakes his head disparagingly and quips, "Marge, it's uter-us, not uter-you." Remember Homer's sage advice should you ever dare have the urge to lay more than half the blame on your wife. As I said a few paragraphs back—your wife needs her *partner* now. An equal, split-down-the-middle, 50-50 partner. One who is as willing to share the credit as he is to share the blame. Anything less is unacceptable. Anything less and you're not even worthy of her.

Respect Her Wishes

Throughout this book, I've stressed a husband's obligation to keep his wife on track and gently nudge her

---

[15]For the record, the next time I sent her flowers was the day we found out our surrogate was pregnant. Now that was the right time.

when she starts to lose steam. But right now, after a failed IVF, you might just want to cool it for a while. Your wife has been through hell. You both have. And if she's now at a place where she wants to take a break or rethink her priorities, then for God's sake, let her do it.

You guys probably went into this thinking that having your own biological child was the be-all and end-all. That anything "less" would be a very distant consolation prize. But that was a lifetime ago now. Opinions may have changed. Attitudes may have changed. Finances have definitely changed. And yesterday's "never in a million years" might be today's "I want it more than anything else in the world."

As I said before: If your resolve is strong enough, you and your wife *will* become parents. It might not happen in the way you originally intended. But, rest assured, it will happen all the same. What follows is a true account of a husband who (along with his wife), made the decision to adopt a child after their second IVF failed. For some couples this is a no-brainer. For others it's a bit more of a hurdle to overcome. For this family, the decision proved a blessing in every possible way.

Tom's Story[16]

Tom is 44 years old and has been married to Alicia for 9 years. They are the parents of a five-year-old girl who was adopted from China.

Tom and Alicia tried a number of ways to get pregnant, but after the second failed IVF, they decided to adopt. Tom said, "The second time we got the news, she completely broke down and was an emotional wreck. Also, the financial burden was huge. That's when I suggested we look at adoption." For him, it wasn't a huge leap: "Whatever road we went down that led us to our daughter—that was the road we were supposed to take." Alicia talked to friends who'd adopted a little girl from China, and after that was absolutely on board.

Tom admits that Alicia still harbors some guilt about not conceiving, but the joy of their daughter far outweighs it. "I'd be naïve to say no, she's over it. But it's certainly not troubled her day-to-day relationship with her child. For us, there's absolutely no difference between our daughter and a biological child. Absolutely none. Other than the way she looks—that's about it."

---

[16]All the names have been changed, more at my request than the husband's.

Tom also offered the following advice for couples who are contemplating adoption. "If you're going down this road—be sure you're in a strong relationship. Because it's a process that needs support for one another. Also, be really open about your feelings with your spouse, and never let her forget you're a part of it. It's terribly painful for the woman when she doesn't get pregnant. She does feel like less of a woman. And it was my job to say—'you're not.'"

12

GOING INTO EXTRA INNINGS: HOW MANY TIMES CAN WE DO THIS SHIT?

There's no finite number of IVF treatments that any given couple can do. For some, one treatment is more than enough. Be it the pain, the stress, the cost, or merely the toll it's taken on their marriage, they would sooner adopt a baby chimp and call it a day then have to go through that saga again. For others, there is no foreseeable end. They will keep on pounding away until their wallet, their bodies, or their marriage finally give out.

I don't have to tell you which category we fell into.

But just because we did so many IVF treatments, doesn't mean we did them all in exactly the same way. My wife, human dynamo that she is, wasn't going to let a silly little diagnosis like "unexplained infertility" prevent her from trying any other variations on the theme that were currently available. For example, around our fourth or fifth treatment (I lose count), my wife decided that we should try a gamete intrafallopian transfer, or GIFT for short.[17] In this procedure, the still unfertilized eggs and sperm are surgically reimplanted *directly* into the fallopian tubes for fertilization (thus bypassing the cervix altogether). Were we the ideal candidates for this procedure? Probably not. Was I completely on board with doing it? Not really. Did it work? No. But at least she was thinking out of the box a little instead of beating the same dead horse over and over. And, as you'll soon see, it's that kind of forward thinking that led us to our tenth and final IVF treatment—and a new term that I hadn't even heard of yet: gestational surrogate.

DR. ROSEN: There is very little data regarding when a couple should stop doing IVF. We have all heard about the couple that conceived on their 12th attempt, but this is very unusual in two ways. One, very, very few people try this often, and two, most of them do not conceive (Marc and his wife notwithstanding). Generically speaking, the odds that a couple will conceive after three or four tries is really quite small.

If I recall, my wife and I were among those couples who were—how shall I put it—"encouraged" to throw in the towel around our fifth or sixth try (before we

---

[17]Don't let the name throw you. This particular "gift" will cost you upwards of 12 grand.

starting seeing Dr. Rosen). So given that we eventually conceived, was that doctor wrong to dissuade us? Not at all. Due to the increasingly low probability of success, he would have been wrong not to dissuade us. Morally, medically, and ethically, he did exactly what he was supposed to. He discussed our options, advised us of the risks, and left the final decision to us—which, as it turned out, was to continue with the IVFs, but explore new ways of doing it.

Obviously, in hindsight, we made the right choice for ourselves. But had that 10th IVF not worked with the surrogate (which was certainly the odds-on favorite), I'm sure history, as well as myself, would be viewing those choices very differently. In the end, and without the aid of a crystal ball, it's up to each individual couple to weigh the financial, medical, and emotional risks for themselves. Going ahead with that fifth IVF was not an easy decision. Going ahead with the sixth, and seventh, and eighth, was even harder. And I guarantee you that, had we not come out of number 10 with a baby, I'd be kicking myself (and perhaps even blaming my wife) for not beginning the adoption process two years earlier.

I wish I had all the answers. I don't. No one does. All anyone can do is "hope for the best, prepare for the worst, and take whatever comes." And if you can't even do that . . . then maybe it is time to move on.

Switching Doctors: Is it Worth it?

In addition to varying our treatments, my wife also made a practice of switching our doctors—to mixed results and with less-than-enthusiastic support on my part. I didn't necessarily think it was a bad idea . . . just a fairly unwarranted one that was based more on frustration than anything else.

As a screenwriter by trade, I can only compare it to switching agents. (See, I knew my real job would come in handy somehow.) Though I'm not proud of it, I used to switch agents quite a bit. (Sorry Caryn, Steve, and especially Susan.) Sometimes it was warranted. They weren't working hard enough for me, or our sensibilities didn't quite jibe. More often than not, I just wasn't getting the work I wanted and figured it must be their fault. And, at least in the case of those three names I just mentioned, I couldn't have been more wrong.

Switching doctors after an unsuccessful fertility treatment is kind of like that. Sure, there might be better doctors out there, or at least ones you get along with better. If that is the case, then, by all means, shop around for someone else. However, if, for no good reason you're just trying to pin your failure on someone else, then you really might want to reconsider.

As I mentioned in the introduction, we went to five different doctors in three different states (and mind you, we were in California, which still has the most progressive and advanced fertility clinics in the nation). So why did we do it? More often than not, it was hearing that some other clinic had something "new," or something "better," which never proved to be the case. And yet each time we switched, it required moving records, a brand-new "breaking-in" period, and an entirely new office staff for us to butter up and kiss the asses of.

So just think twice before you flippantly decide that it can't be *you*, so it must be *them*. Chances are still more than likely it's you.

"But What if the Doctor Drops Us?"

Yeah, it happens. More than you probably want to know. You see, a lot of these guys base their reputation on their success rates. You'll hear your wife talking about it, saying things like, "Oh, he's very good. His success rate is over fifty percent." And while this is probably true, it's a hell of a lot more likely he'll succeed with a 30-year-old trying for the first time than with a 35-year-old trying for the sixth.

It happened to us once. Nice doctor, in fact. We liked him a lot. When we started with him, we were young and eager and healthy. His ideal patients. When we ended with him, it was the consultation for our fourth IVF, and he very politely "suggested" that we might be better served elsewhere. He wasn't discouraging. He was just done.

Listen, it happens. It happens in my business, too. I'm just so impatient that I usually beat them to the punch. So if it happens to you, don't sweat it. It's not that you're a bad craps player. It's just that the table's a bit cold right now, and they wouldn't mind finding a new shooter. Life will go on. And the new guy will be even better. Granted, those words may seem pretty meaningless when you have a hysterical wife beside you—and believe me, I did have a hysterical wife beside me—but that still doesn't make the words any less true.

DR. ROSEN: If you do happen to switch doctors, however, please be sure to send over all your medical records way ahead of time. I hate when a new couple comes in, places a phone book worth of records on my desk, and expects answers right away. I obviously need time to read it all and don't want to miss anything important. As Winston Churchill said, "Those that fail to learn from history are doomed to repeat it."

13

THE CHANGE-UP: EXPLORING OTHER OPTIONS

We were going to China. We had the name of an orphanage. We had started the process. But in the meantime, there were still a few—not many, but a few—more radical and/or controversial treatments left to try.

In this next chapter, I'll talk about some of those treatments, including the one that finally worked for us—gestational surrogacy.

Using a Sperm or Egg Donor

Okay, this is a big one. Not so much physically as emotionally. For the first time in this process, you and your wife may be considering a treatment that will result in a child who is biologically related to only one of you. Some people have trouble with this. My wife and I had trouble with this. As far as we were concerned, no biological connection was better than half. Maybe it was the whole "equal partners" thing. Maybe it was just plain ego. But whatever the reason, this wasn't an option that appealed to us, even if we had been good candidates. For many couples, however, sperm or egg donation is not only a viable option, but a welcome one—especially if it means the wife can still carry her baby to term.

In the old days, sperm donation was the only game in town. Sperm was easy to acquire, easy to freeze, and easy to inseminate. It still is. However, with more and more treatments like ICSI (see chapter 8), the need for donated sperm is becoming less and less prevalent.[18] Donated eggs, on the other hand, are a whole other story—especially now that so many "older" women, with a less-than-ideal egg supply, are trying to get pregnant.

"How Does Egg Donation Work?"

The technology needed for egg donation has been around for only about 20 years, but in that time it has proved a godsend to thousands of childless couples. Unlike sperm, which can be inseminated directly into the cervix via a catheter, donated eggs aren't nearly as

---

[18]Like everything else in this book, my focus is on heterosexual, married couples. Obviously, for lesbian couples or single women (just two examples) sperm donation is still widely used.

easy to procure. In a procedure very similar to your standard IVF, the donor is bombarded with a series of birth control pills, Lupron, and a slew of follicle-stimulating injections to produce as many of her eggs as possible (thus giving you the best bang for your buck). At the same time, your wife must "sync up" her body with the donor's for the eventual transfer. Like the donor, she must take the birth control pills and Lupron, but instead of the shots, she need only take a pill or wear a skin patch that administers the uterus-ripening hormone, estrogen. When the time is right, the donor's eggs are first extracted, then mixed in the petri dish with your sperm, and finally reimplanted into your wife's body for what one can only hope is a successful pregnancy.

"And How Does One Find an Egg Donor?"

Fortunately, egg donors are fairly abundant. It's not like trying to track down a liver or a kidney. Maybe that's because unlike liver or kidney donors, egg donors are actually paid for their biological material, in some cases quite handsomely. I guess, in some ways, that makes the term "donor" a bit of a misnomer, but then again, "egg seller" sounds so crass.

While many couples will begin and end their egg search with their fertility doctor—possibly even finding a donor within their own clinic—I'd strongly encourage seeking out a reputable broker or organization that specializes in egg donation. Not only will these professionals have carefully screened all candidates, but they will also help to negotiate any conflicts and assist with all the legal documentation that, as you can imagine, is pretty voluminous.

"So How Much are Eggs Going for These Days?"

That depends entirely on where you go and what you're looking for. If a friend or relative is willing to lend a hand (or a few eggs as the case may be), then they might cost you nothing. If, on the other hand, you want a blond-haired, blue-eyed donor with an Ivy League education and a flair for the violin, then you could be talking much more—really anything. But, on average, your typical first-rate egg donor is going to charge you in the neighborhood of $7,500. Keep in mind, however, that that still doesn't include the IVF treatment itself, the slew of medications, the legal expenses, and any fee that a broker will (most deservingly) charge. When all is said and done, we could be talking upwards of $35,000!

"But We Can Find a Woman Who Looks Just Like My Wife, Right?"

Yes, to a certain extent you can. Most brokers will present you with a list of potential candidates whose physical characteristics and traits will all be listed in detail. In many cases, you can even see the woman's photograph to better help you make your choice. However, just because the baby *looks* like your wife's biological child, doesn't mean it *is* her biological child—and it's vital that the two of you discuss up front how much of an issue that will be. In other words, who do you tell, when will you explain it to your future child, and how will you handle it once he or she is old enough to understand?

Given that your wife will be carrying, and ultimately delivering, this baby, the argument can certainly be made for telling absolutely no one (except your child, of course) about the egg donor—not even close family and friends. However, before you go pretending this never happened, it's important to consider the stigma, and unfair burden, this may place on your child when he or she finds out. Granted, the decision to use an egg donor is nobody else's business, but by the same token you don't want to make it your family's "dirty little secret" either.

Listen, this is some pretty heady stuff, and unfortunately there's no rulebook to say how you should, or shouldn't, handle it. So just make sure both of you are on the same page before you venture down this road. And by all means, seriously consider other options if you're not.

What follows is a firsthand account from a husband who (along with his wife, of course) conceived their children through egg donation. As you'll see, this is never a decision to be taken lightly, but, by the same token, I've never met a couple who were anything but thrilled that they had made it.

Frank's Story[19]

Frank is 38 years old and has been married to Mindy for eight years. They are the parents of beautiful twin five-year-olds who were conceived through egg donation.

After finding out that Mindy had a very low chance of conceiving naturally (due to poor egg quality), the couple first turned to less traditional methods of getting pregnant, including an herbalist and an acupuncturist, even though the doctor advised against it. Frank, too, had his reservations. "I knew these holistic methods weren't

---

[19]Again, all names changed.

working, but I thought it best to just let her go through it and wait for the other shoe to drop." Which, after about a year, it finally did. I asked Frank about their state of mind at that point. "Extreme anxiety. Not knowing what the next step should be. A lot of confusion. And that caused stress on the marriage." After weighing their available options, Mindy and Frank briefly considered adoption, but chose egg donation instead. "I've always believed in nurture over nature, so I really didn't care which route we chose. Mindy felt much worse about it than I did, because she wasn't going to be a biological parent, so she had huge guilt issues." In the end, maybe because she could carry these babies, it was Mindy's decision to go with donor eggs (which, ultimately, took three attempts to work, all with the same donor). "In addition to the obvious disappointment, the financial burdens were huge. Huge! My mom left me some money when she passed away—not a great deal. We were dipping into that 'trust fund' every time. 'Whoops, there goes another 25 grand.' That money would have been the kids' college fund, but now it's almost gone." I asked Frank how the egg donation process works. "You go through an agency. The agency gives you a bunch of profiles to look at. They have pictures and bios of the women, and you select one or two or three you're interested in; then the agency goes and checks what the availability is, and that's it. I think we wrote a letter to her as well saying we thought she'd be perfect for us and we wanted her egg to make our family." Even though Mindy would not be biologically related to the children (or perhaps because of it), she wanted to find a donor who was physically similar to herself. This, of course, begged the question of who would know about the egg donor, and when they would find out. *"Our families knew everything from the start and were completely supportive. We weren't quite as forthcoming with friends. At least at first. There was a bit of shame and trepidation in discussing this with the outside world. At any level. As we progressed through the journey, though, that became less and less, but some of it still remains today. The fact that we did egg donation isn't something we discuss freely. It's something we're still coming to terms with."* With regard to the kids, Frank and Mindy have not told them yet, but have every intention of doing so now that they are old enough to understand.[20] And

---

[20]This interview was conducted more than a year ago, and I recently called Frank to ask how he went about telling the children, and how they reacted to the news. I was less than surprised to hear that he and Mindy had not yet told them (the twins are already seven years old). This seems to be the case with nearly all of the egg donor couples I have spoken to, which is why I can't stress

what about the donor herself? As is protocol, Frank and Mindy have no contact with her. When asked how he felt about the kids attempting communication as adults, he responded simply yet firmly, "That's not an option." Still, for all that they went through, Frank has absolutely no regrets. "It was extremely stressful. But ultimately I'd say it brought us closer together insofar as we went through a tough challenge and came out the other end intact. I don't think there was much negative about it, except for me having to shoot her up twice a day or whatever it was. It was a rough experience—one I'd rather not have gone through—but the ends definitely justify the means."

Donor Eggs with a Side of Surrogate, Please.

Implanting another woman's eggs not high-tech enough for you? Fear not. For woman who can neither produce viable eggs nor carry to term, an increasingly popular option is to combine the husband's sperm with another woman's eggs (the

---

enough to share this information with them as early as possible (age five probably would have been about right). The longer these couples wait, the harder the conversation will be—both for them and for their children.

donor) and then hire yet another woman (the surrogate) to carry the resulting embryos to term. Many celebrities in their forties and fifties have gone this route, whether they'll admit to using donor eggs or not. It's also a popular option for gay couples, as well as single men who desire children (an oxymoron if ever there was one).

Now why, you might ask, would any couple in their right mind choose to hire two separate women, rather than just have the husband artificially inseminate the egg donor? I mean, isn't that as stupid as when one movie theater employee sells you the ticket and a whole other employee rips it? Actually, it's not, and here's why. Because if the same woman both produces the eggs *and* carries them (in other words, she's both the biological and the birth mother) you do run the risk—however slight—of having her fight for parental custody down the road. A nightmarish scenario that's all but eradicated if you split up the duties between two woman.

Please bear in mind, however, that getting both an egg donor *and* a surrogate is prohibitively expensive and hardly an option for those who don't have their own network TV show.

Embryo Adoption

Hell, who says you have to stop with a donated egg or donated sperm? Why not go ahead and implant the whole damn thing into your wife? Donated embryos usually come from couples who, after a successful (or unsuccessful) IVF treatment, choose to anonymously donate their remaining stock to fellow infertility sufferers like yourselves. Pretty selfless stuff if you ask me. I know I couldn't do it. Be that as it may, this is a great option for couples who (a) might feel funny having a kid who is "more" one partner's than the other, and (b) feel strongly about experiencing a pregnancy. Also, as opposed to a more "traditional" adoption, you've eliminated the risk of a birth mother who suddenly changes her mind.

Immune Therapies

With tongue-twisting names like leukocyte immune therapy and intravenous immunoglobulin, these procedures are so controversial that many aren't even legal in this country. I'm not gonna delve any deeper into this (if for no other reason than I don't understand it), but if you're willing to invest in an overseas phone call,

I'm sure there's some doctor in Belgium who'd love to tell you more.

Gestational Surrogacy

Finally a procedure I don't have to bullshit my way through. For better or worse, I know about this one all too well. Like egg donation, gestational surrogacy requires the participation of a third party, but here's the twist: Instead of taking someone else's eggs and giving them to your wife to carry, your wife's eggs (along with your sperm), are implanted into another woman (the surrogate) for her to carry. The downside is that your wife doesn't get to experience pregnancy (as if any man could really call that a downside), but the upside is that any resulting children are 100 percent biologically hers and yours. Of course, it's not like you can just "choose" gestational surrogacy over egg donation (or vice versa). It all depends on what's causing your infertility problems in the first place. For example, if you and your wife produce perfect embryos but none ever take, then a gestational surrogate may be a viable option. If, on the other hand, your wife's reproductive system is perfectly fine, but her eggs are not, then an egg donor would probably make more sense.

Which is yet another reason why "unexplained infertility" is such a frustrating diagnosis.

Truth be told, no doctor ever recommended that we try gestational surrogacy. In fact, many discouraged it. The prevailing wisdom was this: If a woman's infertility cannot be diagnosed, then chances are more than likely her eggs are at fault—in which case, hiring another woman to carry them would prove futile. My wife, on the other hand, believed differently. Throughout all of our IVFs, she had no problem producing eggs, and our resulting embryos were always good. It was only when they were placed back in her body that things fell apart. To her mind (and, at the time, her mind only), this meant that the fault must lie somewhere within her own reproductive system. In fact, she had started investigating gestational surrogacy long before we actually tried it, and, if not for the discouragement of the doctors (and myself to some degree), we might have even explored it earlier.

I tell you this to stress a point that I've made a few times in this book. Nobody knows your wife's body better than she does. And while science is great, and doctors are invaluable, you should also (a) never discount the power of some good old common sense, (b) never be afraid to "think outside the box," and

(c) never, I repeat, never, ignore the gut feelings of a woman on a mission. If I had only listened to her sooner, we probably could have avoided IVFs seven, eight, and nine altogether.

Finding a Surrogate

Like egg donors, gestational surrogates can be found through a number of different sources—family and friends, personal ads, and professional brokers being the most common routes. We used an organization called the Center for Surrogate Parenting (CSP) in Los Angeles, and I couldn't recommend them more highly. They were as caring, thorough, and professional as you would demand a service of this nature to be.

Now, here's the good news about gestational surrogates. They need not be young, nubile 25-year-olds. Unlike egg donors, who are giving you a part of their bodily material, a gestational surrogate is little more than a human oven; so long as she is in good health and capable of carrying a child, she is a viable candidate. That's why you might have even heard of mothers being gestational surrogates for their daughter's babies.

Here's the bad news: Compared with egg donors, gestational surrogates aren't nearly as easy to come by. In fact, when we first went to CSP, there was only about one surrogate for every ten wanting couples. It's just not that easy to find a really qualified woman who's willing to give up nine months of her life to carry someone else's baby.

So why would any sane person do it, you might ask? Well, certainly there's the money. About $30,000 on average. But for most women, the financial compensation is hardly the motivating factor. Our own surrogate put it this way: "It's the closest I could ever come to being an angel."

I don't believe in heaven. I don't believe in hell. But I do believe that woman is an angel. She will always be our angel.

"Very sweet. But how much does this shit cost?"

A lot. Between the IVF itself, all the medication, the legal fees, the broker fees, and the surrogate's well-earned 30 large, you're probably looking at somewhere in the neighborhood of $75,000 to $100,000 dollars. I know. That's insane. But miracles don't come cheap.

"So how does gestational surrogacy work?"

Well, as I alluded to before, unless you've got a really nice sister-in-law with a shitload of time on her hands, the hardest part of gestational surrogacy will be finding the surrogate in the first place. Remember, surrogacy is the only procedure that actually requires the day-to-day participation of a third party. You're not just dealing indirectly or anonymously with another woman. You're potentially handing your kid(s) over to a virtual stranger for the better part of a year!

Without getting into all the details of the matching process, suffice it to say that we got lucky. Our surrogate (along with her husband) was the first one we met, and the connection was immediate. The only potential drawback was that they lived more than 300 miles away, in Northern California, but thankfully this never presented a problem.

Once our connection was established and we agreed to work together, the next step was to sync up the surrogate's cycle with my wife's. In many ways, this was like all our other IVF treatments, except at the final stage of transfer, the embryos (four of them) were placed in the surrogate's body instead of my wife's. The other plus to this was that my wife was now off the hook for those dreaded progesterone shots, and, as it turned out, she was also off the hook for the even more dreaded and uncomfortable task of carrying twins.

"Weren't you afraid she'd steal the babies?"

My wife and I got asked that one a lot. To be honest, we asked it ourselves at our first meeting with CSP—and the answer they gave us was this: In all their years of doing this, never, not once, had a surrogate ever "run off" with a couple's babies or attempted to keep them after the birth. In fact, the only thing that had happened a time or two was that the couple—because of a pending divorce or a natural pregnancy—decided halfway through the process that they didn't want their babies anymore, thus leaving this poor surrogate to deliver a child (or children) that would then have to be put up for adoption. So, if anything, the surrogate need be more leery of the couple than the couple of the surrogate.

Given that everyone's experiences are bound to be different, here's a firsthand account from another husband who also went through gestational surrogacy with his wife—and used the wife's sister as their surrogate!

Dave's Story[21]

Dave is 45 years old and has been married to Lynn (44) for 10 years. They have one son (Sam) who is 7 years old and was born through a gestational surrogate (Lynn's sister, who was married with two small children).

After a series of miscarriages and two unsuccessful IVFs (due to a problem with Lynn's uterus) she and Dave briefly considered adoption but elected to try gestational surrogacy first. Lynn's sister quickly volunteered, and despite Dave's initial hesitation, they moved forward. "The sister aspect, to me, was problematic. I would have much preferred using a surrogate from the agency. Those people seemed lovely. Doing it altruistically—wanting to be an angel—I thought this was good. But then Lynn said, 'My sister can do it,' and I thought this could lead to huge problems. Huge problems. What if something went wrong? Would one sister blame the other forever? If it was a stranger, they would do it and go away, but an aunt's going to be in your life forever. Is that going to be weird, is that going to be difficult? I had all these misgivings about it."

Thankfully, Dave's misgivings proved unfounded, in no small part because he (smartly) insisted that,

---

[21]As you might have guessed by now, all names changed.

family or not, they go about this as officially as possible. "I sat down with them. I said let's talk about this. Two things: First, if we do this, we need to go through the surrogacy center so there's an intermediary; there are a lot of people that don't do that. Second, you have to go through their tests to make sure you're fit—physically, mentally, all those things—are you willing to do that? Yes. Okay. I also wanted to pay all the expenses through the surrogacy center so she wouldn't feel awkward about asking and we wouldn't feel awkward about paying. Okay. Fine. Finally, everybody has to agree that if something goes horribly wrong—if we lose babies—no one will be blamed. Or if something physically happens to her sister during birth—I mean, this is risky. It's birth."[22]

Still, despite every attempt to the contrary, it was inevitable that some small issues would arise, mostly to do with Lynn's sister refusing help or not accepting maternity clothes and other necessities. "I had to settle fights between people. I had to sometimes throw money at things and stop things from going in bad directions. I

---

[22]There is obviously no way to guarantee that no one will be blamed and, in fact, had something gone dreadfully wrong, it's more than likely someone would have. Still, the more information communicated (and written down), the better. This is the last place you want assumptions and misunderstandings and hearsay.

had to pull my wife over and say 'Let it go'—and take a stand about giving her sister space. Or say 'Let's do this regardless of what your sister says—and then let's move forward.'"

I asked Dave about Lynn's sister's family—how they all dealt with this pregnancy that, in many ways, was not their own. "The kids (ages 2 and 4) always knew it was Aunt Lynn's baby. They totally got it. Even now, Lynn's sister treats my child no differently from any of her other nephews. There's no uncomfortableness or weirdness. We thanked her. We gave her a tummy tuck. She didn't want anything else. When it's our son's birthday, we call and thank her—but it really has faded away. We don't favor her in any other way." And what about other people— friends and other family members—how much did they know about all this? "We decided early on, first, it's going to be the history of this baby and the baby's gonna know its history, and second, to properly give credit where credit is due. To make my sister-in-law feel loved and appreciated, it also helps to tell everybody, 'Look what this woman's doing—it's fantastic.' This isn't to say we announced it to anyone who would listen, but we wouldn't lie about it, either. If someone at a party asked how Lynn was feeling, I would simply say, 'Well actually, she's not carrying the baby.' And then take it from there." And what about their *now seven-year-old son? Were they just as forthcoming with him? "Of course. We told him as soon as he could understand. We saw no other option. At first we would just say 'Mommy's tummy was broken,' but at this age he knows more about biology—egg, sperm, DNA."*

In total, Dave and Lynn, like my wife and me, spent about a quarter of a million dollars on their fertility treatments—about a third of that for the gestational surrogacy (he claims to have saved nothing by using a relative, given that they still worked through an agency). The couple have since tried to get pregnant again, both with Lynn's sister and professional gestational surrogates, but have thus far been unsuccessful. "I wanted to go ahead and have a second child much quicker. Our son was born, and six months later I'm ready to start again. We'd have two kids close in age—done with diapers. Family trips become this and that. No, she wants to be a mother to him first. So by the time she wants to try also, it's three or four years later. Lynn was older. The eggs were older. The surrogates weren't as fertile as we hoped. Who knows? The surrogate got pregnant a couple of times and miscarried. Eventually, I pulled the trigger and said 'I'm stopping. I've had enough.' Every time we got pregnant and every time there was a miscarriage, it was a heartbreaking experience. The whole process is so time-consuming.

It's draining. I said, 'I'm done. I can't do it.' We tried a couple of years. I'm happy with my boy. I'm thrilled to be a dad."

I then asked if Lynn was as content about the situation as he was. "Not for about a year. She said, 'I'm not ready.' Okay—we'll try one more time. I listened. Later, I said 'I am done. I know you're not ready—but I am done. You want to get a donor, fine, but I'm not doing it.' We still talk about it. It's still a possibility. But our son is seven now. My preference was for kids a little closer in age. It'd almost be like two families. I'm thrilled to not be worried about it. We investigated adoption, but it's the opposite of what we experienced with surrogacy. The women seem pretty selfless in surrogacy; in adoption they seemed more selfish. It's all about what you can do for them— then they'll give you the baby. The process is a lot less open and giving, at least in our experience."

With all of this now behind them, I wondered how their relationship had changed, either for better or worse. "Like all tests, it makes you stronger. It brings you together. To have a common bond of trying to get pregnant is a prelude to the common bond of parenting— which is like insane glue. If you're both on the same track about parenting, you can forget about everything else. You're just like one machine. It certainly was an entrée to that." So, looking back, what did Dave learn from all this, and what might he have done differently? "If anything, I wish I had been less resistant going in. I'd have gone straight to IVF. Why waste the money and the time when all the signs are already pointing there? Ultimately, the hardest thing, at least for me, was remembering that 'this too shall pass.' Pregnancy is all encompassing, but when the baby comes—who gives a shit how it was born? Really. It's just a little bit of history and that's it."

14

SUCCESS AT LAST!

July 2, 2002. It was during our "twelve days from hell." Our agreed upon *last* twelve days from hell, regardless of the outcome. By now I pretty much had the drill down pat. Stay out of her way, listen when she spoke, try to get her mind off it as best I could. We were at the Santa Monica Pier. A futile diversion that I thought might pass the time. Instead, it was just an ongoing discussion of why my wife thought it was a good idea to check in with the surrogate for the umpteenth time, and why I thought it wasn't. Of course, she won out.

So in a parking lot by the beach I picked up my cell phone and dialed. And shortly into the conversation, the surrogate dropped the bombshell. "I know I wasn't supposed to, but I took a pregnancy test. Actually, three pregnancy tests." My heart sank. My wife looked on with curiosity. I moved a few steps away. "And . . . ?" "And they were all positive." At first the words didn't even register. Six years of failure will tend to have that effect on you. I took a breath and asked how she thought I should break the news. She repeated the results . . . and this time it clicked. (See Fig. 3 for the picture she later sent us.)

Let me stress it again: You and your wife *will* become parents. It might not be now, and it might not be in the way you intended, but one way or another, if your resolve is strong enough, it will happen.

Now, would it suck if you went through even a third of what we did, only to wind up at the adoption agency you could have just gone to in the first place? Yes and

Fig. 3: A Picture's Worth a Thousand Words

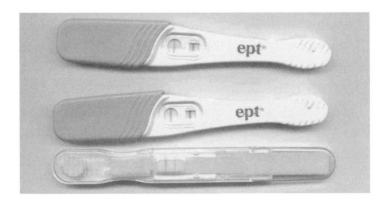

no. I mean, granted—your money could have been a hell of a lot better spent on a new Porsche Carerra than it could on a bunch of failed in vitros. But the truth is, you might have needed those failed in vitros to bring you to a place where the adoption finally felt right.

As I told you in the beginning of the book . . . it's a process.

My process, or my journey if you will, led me through three states, five doctors, and, finally, to a parking lot in Santa Monica, California, where I made the most wonderful and memorable phone call of my life. Yours may lead you as close as your nearest pharmacy, or as far away as Russia or China.[23] There's really no way of knowing.

But what I do know is this: When you get there . . . in that moment . . . everything you did before will all seem worth it. I promise you it will.

---

[23]Foreign adoptions are becoming increasingly popular these days, with China and Russia being two of the most common, and most in-demand, destinations for perspective parents.

PART FOUR
THE POSTGAME ANALYSIS

There was a lot of stuff to cover in this book. And while I tried my best to make it as coherent and straightforward as possible, you couldn't be expected to remember all of it. So, if nothing else, here's a quick "highlight reel" of the five most important points to remember:

1. Communicate

Always the most important thing. You can't know what your wife wants or needs unless you keep those lines of communication open. And this applies to everything—from when you should start treatments, to who you should tell, to how long you should keep it up.

2. Empathize

Don't just sympathize. Empathize. The last thing your wife needs is pity. You have to show her that you're *feeling* her pain as well.

3. Set unbreakable goals . . . and be ready to break them

Conviction is great. A single-minded plan is great. But you have to be willing to shift gears as the situation warrants, and you have to make sure your wife is willing to as well.

4. Never stand on ceremony

Simply cast aside any stubbornness or machismo you might have if it in any way interferes with the goal. Don't want to take a semen analysis test? Too bad. Feel uncomfortable discussing your personal life with a doctor? Get over it. Infertility is demoralizing, invasive, and messy. That's just the way is. Sorry.

5. Share the burden

As easy as it might be to sit back and let your wife do all the work, it is perhaps the worst decision you could ever make. You *can* be useful in this process. In fact, you can be indispensable. Please don't let that opportunity pass you by.

If you've gotten this far in the book, congratulations. If you merely skipped to the back, don't sweat it. Those five points pretty much sum up the whole thing anyway.

Listen, infertility is tough. And anyone who hasn't been through it couldn't even begin to understand how tough it really is. I've been through it. I understand it all too well. And from the bottom of my heart I wish you all the luck in the world.

AFTERWORD

On September 9, 2005, I witnessed another miracle. At exactly 12:57 PM, my third child, Michael Emerson Sedaka, was born. A beautiful baby boy—weighing in at a robust eight pounds—had just gasped his first breath.

This, however, was not the miracle.

The miracle was that the woman who delivered my son—a near-perfect combination of both me and my wife—*was*, in fact, my wife. An infertile woman who had proven time and time again that she couldn't carry a baby to term had, amazingly, done just that.

A completely natural conception, a trouble-free pregnancy, a textbook birth.

So, in the end, we wound up becoming that cliché—the couple who couldn't have a baby on their own, finally doing so through artificial means, and then, when the pressure was off, suddenly getting knocked up when they weren't even trying.

Tell that one to your wife the next time she insists that stress doesn't play a part.

INDEX